Program Evaluation For Healthcare Systems & Educational Programs

Dr. Lisa Marie Portugal, PhD, EdD
The Leadership Architect

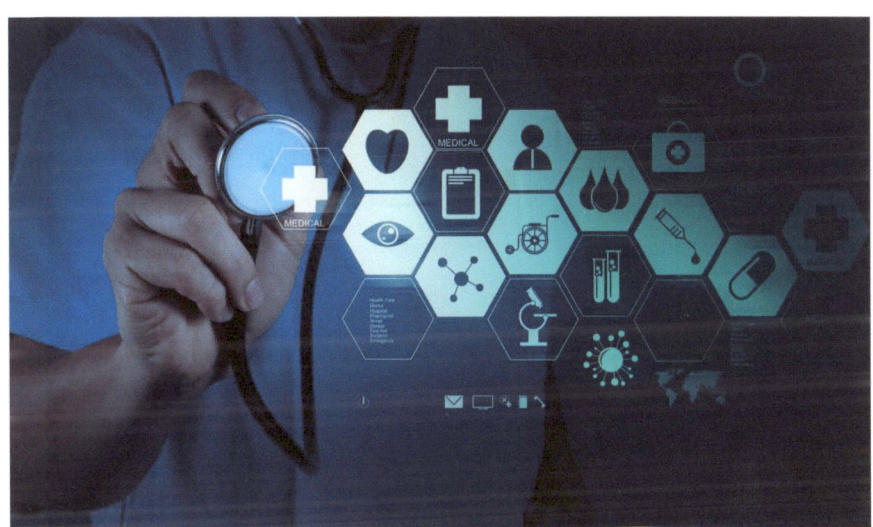

**Program Evaluation
For Healthcare Systems & Educational Programs**

Copyright © August 16, 2017 by Dr. Lisa Marie Portugal, PhD, EdD
All rights reserved under copyright conventions.
Published in the United States by Dr. Lisa Marie Portugal, PhD, EdD
The Leadership Architect

Library of Congress Cataloguing-in-Publication data is available
ISBN 978-1974108169
Printed in the United States
First Edition

Table of Contents

Back Cover Text	5
Introduction	7
Evaluation & Assessment	10
Framework for Program Evaluation in Public Health	17
Assembling an Evaluation Team	21
Logic Modeling in Program Evaluation	39
Decision-Oriented Approach or the CIPP Model	42
SMART goals	47
Approaches to Conducting an Audit	51
Guiding Principles of Evaluation	53
The Evaluator's Role	57
Effective Evaluation Models	58
Ethics Self-Assessment	61
Purpose & Logic Model	63
Evaluation Design	71
Data Collection	74
Comparing & Contrasting Qualitative & Quantitative	80
Reliability, Validity, & Ethics	85
Data Analysis & Interpretation	98
Qualitative Research Approaches to Program Evaluation	100
Use, Communication, & Evaluation	108
Template Using Quantitative & Qualitative Approaches	112
Logic Model Charts	119
American College of Healthcare Code of Ethics	125
Conclusion	132
Appendix	133
About the Author	141
Contact	143
References	145
Disclaimer	151

Back Cover Text

Leaders regularly engage in evaluation of programs, processes, and structures to identify their relative efficacy and determine changes that might be needed. Fitzpatrick (2004) notes that qualitative and quantitative methods be used cooperatively in program evaluation given that "diverse frameworks offer a richness of perspectives... especially if one uses evaluation approaches eclectically." This book compares and contrasts the underlying philosophy, assumptions, and components of quantitative and qualitative approaches to program evaluation. In addition, a description of how one might design a program evaluation employing a combination of quantitative and qualitative approaches is examined for professionals and leaders in health-related occupations.

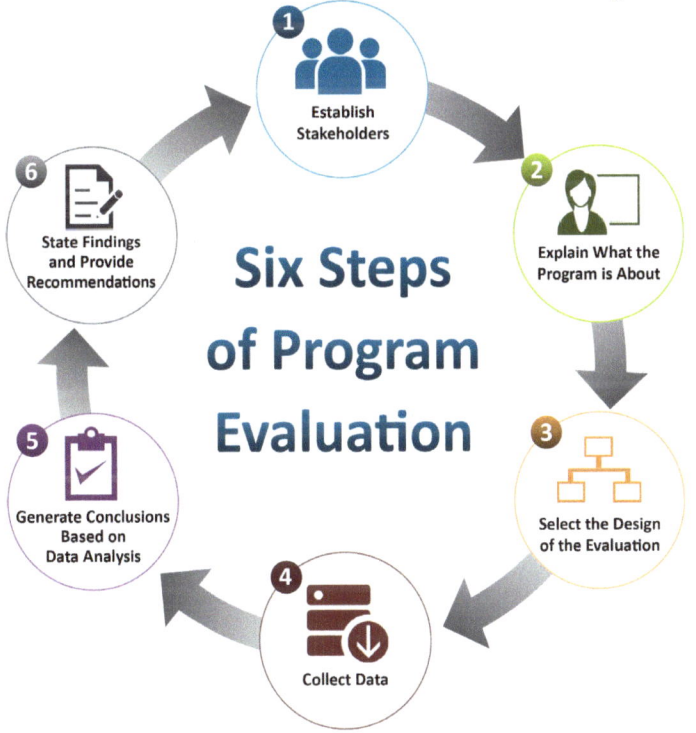

Introduction

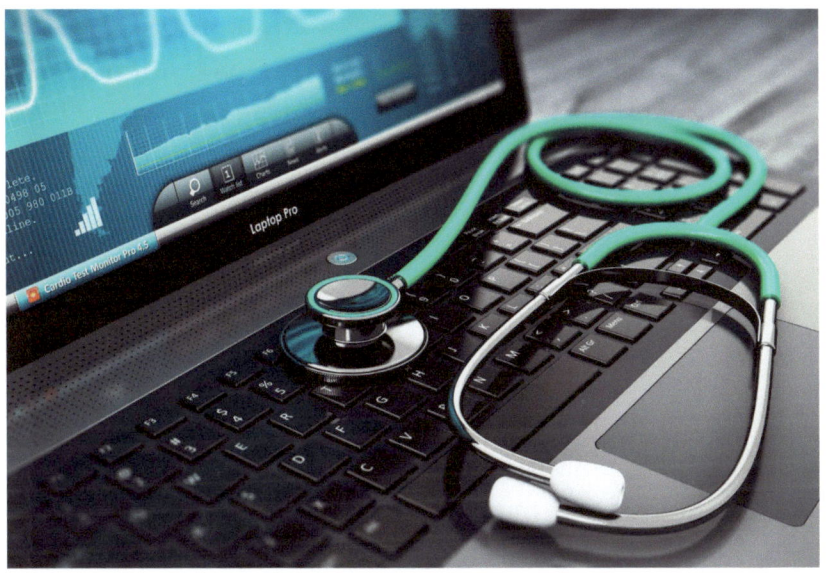

This book provides an example of how one might design a program evaluation of a health care system or education program. In addition, how to outline an evaluation and what components are involved based upon standard program evaluation methods are presented. The meaning of qualitative and quantitative research as identified by the literature is interpreted. Finally, underlying philosophy, assumptions, and components of quantitative and qualitative approaches to program evaluation is compared and contrasted with an appendix template provided.

This book will:

- Explain assessment and evaluation processes.
- Describe the benefits of program evaluation and its application in healthcare education and clinical settings.
- Analyze the impact of Bloom's Taxonomy, SMART goals, and other factors on learning, assessment, and evaluation.
- Compare and contrast theoretical frameworks, designs, or models for evaluation
- Explain the role of reliability, validity, and ethics in the evaluation process.
- Describe the importance of communicating assessment and evaluation expectations.
- Relate evaluation to ongoing, continuous improvement in healthcare programs.

Quantitative & Qualitative Research Approaches to Program Evaluation

According to Rao and Woolcock (2003), both qualitative and quantitative approaches incorporated into one's program evaluation adds richness, depth, and strength to one's assessment rather than using only one method, which can be limiting. In addition, by integrating both methods in one's evaluation, there will be less room for researcher bias, assumption, or prejudgment of data. Furthermore, by incorporating a mixed method approach, one may be surprised by the data, which may reveal new information or unexpected discovery.

Quantitative Research Approaches to Program Evaluation Philosophy, Assumptions, & Components

Quantitative approaches in program evaluation "permit generalizations to be made about large populations on the basis of much smaller (representative) samples" (Rao and Woolcock, 2003, p. 165). Moreover, a quantitative approach allows other researchers the opportunity to reproduce the same conditions found in one's evaluation to replicate a similar outcome, thereby validating the original findings. Furthermore, by collecting data in numerical form, and by being removed from the original subjects, one can analyze and interpret data which researchers claim upholds rigorous research standards that are empirical, objective, and impartial. The three typical types of quantitative methods include surveys, experiments, and quasi-experiments. According to Gall, Gall, and Borg (2003), quantitative research designs are classified as experimental or nonexperimental. Phenomena are studied as they exist in a nonexperimental design, and in contrast, experimental designs "involve researcher intervention" (Gall, Gall, & Borg, 2003, p. 298). Nonexperimental designs are correlational, descriptive, and causal-comparative.

Table 1
Underlying Assumptions of Quantitative Methods

Reality is objective, independent from the researcher, can be studied objectively;
Researcher is separate and removed from those being researched;
Research is value-free, values of the researcher are not part of the research;
Research is constructed on deduction, logic, theories, and hypotheses, research is tested in a cause and effect manner; and
Quantitative methods seek to develop generalizations contributing to theory enabling the researcher to understand a particular phenomenon, explain, or predict.

From "A Judge's Deskbook on the Basic Philosophies and Methods of Science: Model Curriculum," by S. A. Dobbin and S. I. Gatowski, 1999.

Evaluation and Assessment

The Purpose of...

assessment is to **INCREASE** quality.

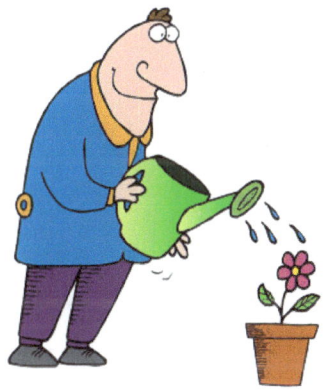

evaluation is to **JUDGE** quality.

Too short and not enough leaves. C-

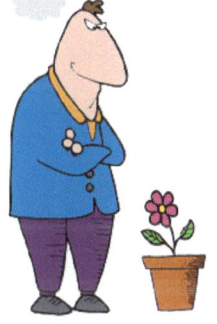

Evaluation and assessment are two different and essential practices that are used to understand outcomes of health and wellness education programs and established systems of health care. Often, the terms assessment and evaluation are used interchangeably. Although both are concerned with quality and performance, they are two complementary but distinct processes. Assessment and evaluation vary in their timing, primary purpose, focus, users, and uses.

Assessment is learner-focused and used to collect data for the purpose of improving the quality of future learner performances. It measures learner progress toward goals or outcomes. Ask these questions, "How well did the learner meet the goals and outcomes? What should I change or modify to improve the outcomes?"

More of an umbrella concept, evaluation is program-focused and used to collect data to measure the quality of present performance. It is judgmental because its ultimate goal is to enable decision making about a program. Ask the questions, "How well did the program meet the goals or outcomes? Should the program continue or be modified?" The key is to recognize how the terms evaluation and assessment are used within a given context. It is important to know how a course, program, or institution is being evaluated or assessed as it changes the perspective of how a measuring instrument is being used.

Perhaps similarities in the processes contribute to the confusion surrounding them. Educator Marie Baehr notes these similarities in assessment and evaluation. Both specify criteria for the purpose of observing a performance or outcome. Used to collect data and evidence, both require a performer, an evaluator or assessor, and a report of findings. Both may be formative (occurring as the performance takes place) or summative (after the performance is completed).

Differences in process occur in the relationships between the performer and the evaluator or assessor. In assessment, the focus of control rests with the performer. In evaluation, it rests with the evaluator. Reports to the performer are also different. In assessment, no mention of quality is made – only references to the strength of the performance and how it could be improved. In evaluation, only information about the quality of the performance is given in the form of a score, grade, or comment. An evaluative report is not used to suggest improvements in future performances.

In the field of healthcare, educational programs are established based on the needs of a target population.

Although the term assessment is used, a needs assessment is actually an evaluation instrument. It is used to determine if a problem or issue exists and to make recommendations for ways to reduce the problem by implementing interventions. A needs assessment is a tool that can be used to: (1) evaluate if a problem or issue exists, (2) examine how a problem might be reduced through interventions, (3) examine whether a program is needed, (4) explore whether a program should be implemented, and (5) evaluate whether the current model in practice should be adapted, altered, revised, or replaced.

The need is identified by collecting and analyzing data. Measurable goals and outcomes are then established to explain how the program will meet the identified need. Goals and outcomes are then aligned to specific criteria or standards. Activities and strategies are selected, and then during implementation, assessments are used to measure progress and meeting the goals and outcomes. In short, a needs assessment tool is used when evaluating existing programs to address: (1) Is the program meeting the identified need? (2) Is the program valuable and worthwhile to the target population? and (3) Should the program be discontinued, continued, modified, or expanded? Evaluation plays a critical role in making these types of determinations.

According to Hays (2009):
> With the expansion of learning in primary care, it naturally follows that more assessment should happen in primary care, for two reasons. One is that primary care is a better source of an increasing range of suitable assessment material, and the other is that 'assessment drives learning'. This means that the increase in core learning in primary care should be reinforced by an increased contribution to core assessment. The assessment role in primary care is therefore increasing in importance. (p. 1)

According to Hays (2009):
> **ASSESSMENT METHODS**
> Methods of clinical assessment form the final part of this paper because there are several methods and the choice will largely be made by the relevant medical school, foundation school or college, as determined by the content of the assessment, as well as the educational impact, validity, reliability and feasibility.9,10 Broadly speaking, there are two formats for clinical assessment: that which is done in controlled circumstances at an examination centre, usually Objective Structured Clinical Examinations (OSCEs) or similar; and workplace-based assessments, where encounters with real patients are assessed in the practice. The latter is where much of the recent development has

focused, as it is arguably a better way to assess for both formative and summative purposes.11 Examples of workplace-based assessment include MSF, case-based orals (CBO), Mini-Clinical Examination (Mini CEx), Mini-Peer Assessment Tool (Mini-PAT) and Direct Observation of Practical Skills (DOPS);12 these are usually observed face to face, but there may be videotape or web-cam alternatives. Other methods include audits of prescribing, referring and record-keeping activity, all particularly important for more senior learners. (p. 6)

Why are assessment and evaluation necessary for clinical positions?

Assessment and evaluation is necessary for clinical positions to improve healthcare quality. Clinical performance relates to the ability of health professionals to apply their knowledge competently in the care of patients or clients. Clinical performance measurement has become foundational to improvement of healthcare quality. Moreover, fair and reasonable evaluation of clinical performance can prove quite challenging.

What challenges may arise in assessing and evaluating clinical personnel?

Fair and reasonable evaluation of clinical performance can be quite challenging and complex. Challenges might include: (1) the evaluation of students, (2) the evaluation of practitioners, (3) skills to be evaluated, (4) accurate assessment and treatment of patients or clients, and (5) the use of appropriate communication tools required to be an effective caregiver.

Other challenges and areas of consideration include: (1) critical thinking skills, (2) ability to maintain appropriate demeanor, (3) ability to prioritize problems, (4) appropriate interactions with others, (5) basic knowledge of clinical procedures, and (6) the ability to complete care procedures correctly. Furthermore, decreasing the anxiety of the practitioner or student being evaluated is also an important factor. In addition, participants, timing, evaluation access and privacy, feedback, and legal and ethical implications should be considered. Finally, per the Family Educational Rights and Privacy Act (FERPA), written performance information must be stored in a secure place. The legal issues relating to the Health Insurance Portability and Accountability Act (HIPAA) are additional considerations in clinical performance evaluation.

Other challenges might include:
1. Evaluator subjectivity and inconsistency,
2. A need to strive for consistency and fairness,
3. The use of a variety of different evaluation tools and strategies such as observation, anecdotal notes, checklists, rating scales, videotapes,
4. The use of written communication, charting, patient progress notes, care plans, process recordings, concept maps, written tests, web-based strategies, clinical conferences, case discussions, and
5. Evaluator awareness of these factors.

FRAMEWORK FOR PROGRAM EVALUATION IN PUBLIC HEALTH

This report presents a framework for understanding program evaluation and facilitating integration of evaluation throughout the public health system. The purposes of this report are to:

- summarize the essential elements of program evaluation;
- provide a framework for conducting effective program evaluations;
- clarify the steps in program evaluation;
- review standards for effective program evaluation; and
- address misconceptions regarding the purposes and methods of program evaluation. (CDC, 1999)

ASSIGNING VALUE TO PROGRAM ACTIVITIES

Assigning value and making judgments regarding a program on the basis of evidence requires answering the following questions:

- What will be evaluated? (That is, what is the program and in what context does it exist?)
- What aspects of the program will be considered when judging program performance?
- What standards (i.e., type or level of performance) must be reached for the program to be considered successful?
- What evidence will be used to indicate how the program has performed?

- What conclusions regarding program performance are justified by comparing the available evidence to the selected standards?
- How will the lessons learned from the inquiry be used to improve public health effectiveness? (CDC, 1999)

FRAMEWORK FOR PROGRAM EVALUATION IN PUBLIC HEALTH

The steps are as follows:

Step 1: Engage stakeholders.
Step 2: Describe the program.
Step 3: Focus the evaluation design.
Step 4: Gather credible evidence.
Step 5: Justify conclusions.
Step 6: Ensure use and share lessons learned.
(CDC, 1999)

The second element of the framework is a set of 30 standards for assessing the quality of evaluation activities, organized into the following four groups:

Standard 1: utility,
Standard 2: feasibility,
Standard 3: propriety, and
Standard 4: accuracy. (CDC, 1999)

Steps in Program Evaluation

Step 1: Engaging Stakeholders

- Those Involved in Program Operations.
- Those Served or Affected by the Program.
- Primary Users of the Evaluation. (CDC, 1999)

Step 2: Describing the Program

- Need
- Expected Effects
- Activities
- Resources
- Stage of Development
- Context
- Logic Model (CDC, 1999)

Step 3: Focusing the Evaluation Design

- Purpose
- Users
- Uses
- Questions
- Methods
- Agreements (CDC, 1999)

Step 4: Gathering Credible Evidence

- Indicators
- Sources
- Quantity

- Quality
- Logistics (CDC, 1999)

Step 5: Justifying Conclusions

- Standards
- Analysis and Synthesis
- Interpretation
- Judgments
- Recommendations. (CDC, 1999)

Step 6: Ensuring Use and Sharing Lessons Learned

- Design
- Preparation
- Feedback
- Follow-Up
- Dissemination
- Additional Uses (CDC, 1999)

Standards for Effective Evaluation

Standards are grouped into the following four categories and include a total of 30 specific standards:

- utility,
- feasibility,
- propriety, and
- accuracy. (CDC, 1999)

APPLYING THE FRAMEWORK

Conducting Optimal Evaluations

Public health professionals can no longer question whether to evaluate their programs; instead, the appropriate questions are:

- What is the best way to evaluate?
- What is being learned from the evaluation? And,
- How will lessons learned from evaluations be used to make public health efforts more effective and accountable? (CDC, 1999)

Assembling an Evaluation Team

A leader must be designated to coordinate the team and maintain continuity throughout the process; thereafter, the steps in evaluation practice guide the selection of team members. For example:

- Those who are diplomatic and have diverse networks can engage other stakeholders and maintain involvement.
- When describing the program, persons are needed who understand the program's history, purpose, and practical operation in the field. In addition, those with group facilitation skills might be asked to help elicit unspoken expectations regarding the program and to expose hidden values that partners bring to the effort. Such facilitators can also help the stakeholders create logic models that describe

the program and clarify its pattern of relationships between means and ends.
- Decision makers and others who guide program direction can help focus the evaluation design on questions that address specific users and uses. They can also set logistic parameters for the evaluation's scope, time line, and deliverables.
- Scientists, particularly social and behavioral scientists, can bring expertise to the development of evaluation questions, methods, and evidence gathering strategies. They can also help analyze how a program operates in its organizational or community context.
- Trusted persons who have no particular stake in the evaluation can ensure that participants' values are treated fairly when applying standards, interpreting facts, and reaching justified conclusions.
- Advocates, clear communicators, creative thinkers, and members of the power structure can help ensure that lessons learned from the evaluation influence future decision-making regarding program strategy. (CDC, 1999)

FIGURE 1. Recommended framework for program evaluation

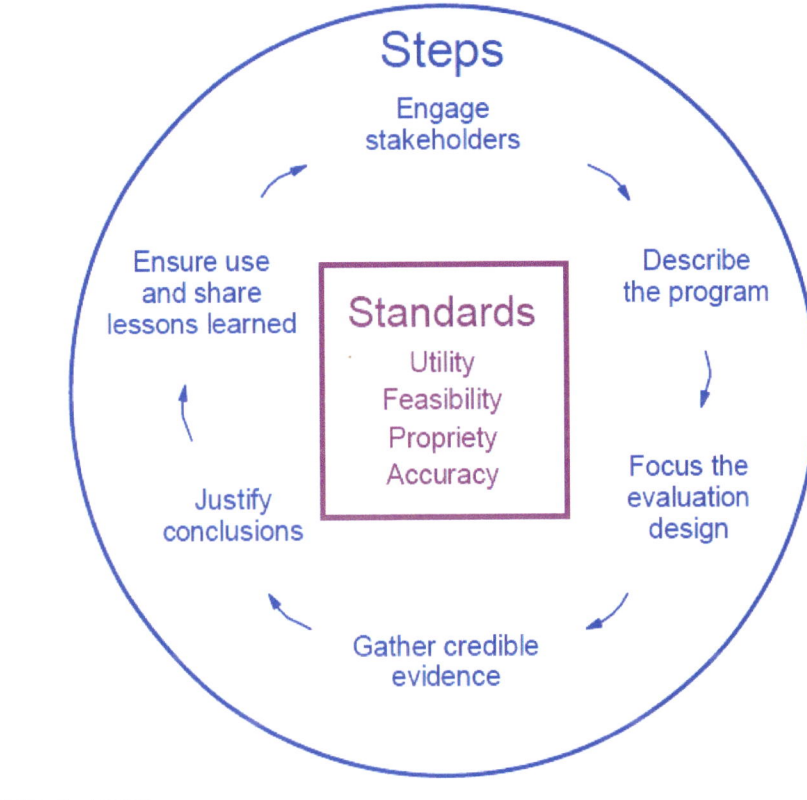

(CDC, 1999)

FIGURE 2. Logic model for a tuberculosis control program

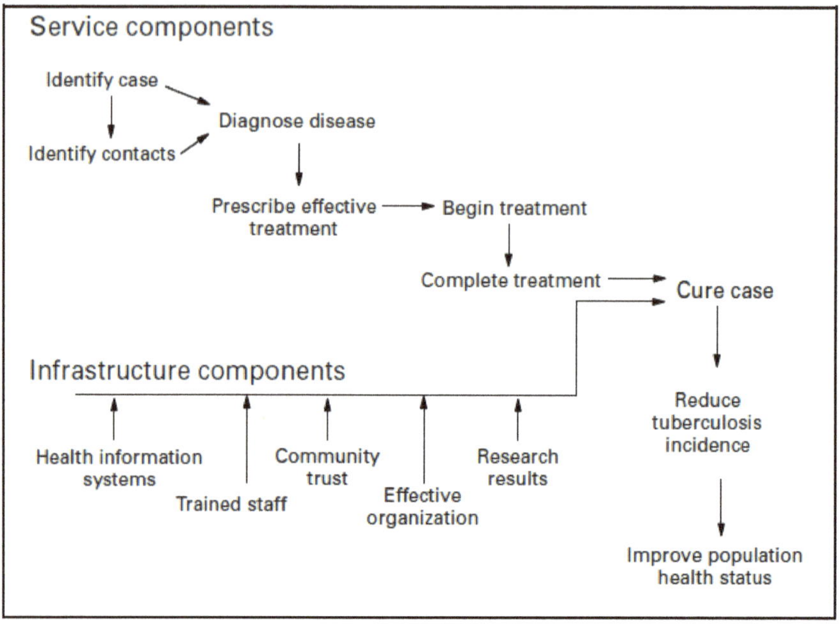

Service components

Identify case → Diagnose disease
Identify contacts → Diagnose disease
Identify case → Identify contacts

Diagnose disease → Prescribe effective treatment → Begin treatment → Complete treatment → Cure case

Infrastructure components

Health information systems, Trained staff, Community trust, Effective organization, Research results

Cure case → Reduce tuberculosis incidence → Improve population health status

(CDC, 1999)

Example Activities

- Characterizing the need (or set of needs) addressed by the program;
- Listing specific expectations as goals, objectives, and criteria for success;
- Clarifying why program activities are believed to lead to expected changes;
- Drawing an explicit logic model to illustrate relationships between program elements and expected changes;
- Assessing the program's maturity or stage of development;
- Analyzing the context within which the program operates;

- Considering how the program is linked to other ongoing efforts; and
- Avoiding creation of an overly precise description for a program that is under development. (CDC, 1999)

Selected uses for evaluation in public health practice by category of purpose:

Gain Insight

- Assess needs, desires, and assets of community members.
- Identify barriers and facilitators to service use.
- Learn how to describe and measure program activities and effects. (CDC, 1999)

Change Practice

- Refine plans for introducing a new service.
- Characterize the extent to which intervention plans were implemented.
- Improve the content of educational materials.
- Enhance the program's cultural competence.
- Verify that participants' rights are protected.
- Set priorities for staff training.
- Make midcourse adjustments to improve patient/client flow.
- Improve the clarity of health communication messages.
- Determine if customer satisfaction rates can be improved.

- Mobilize community support for the program. (CDC, 1999)

Assess Effects

- Assess skills development by program participants.
- Compare changes in provider behavior over time.
- Compare costs with benefits.
- Find out which participants do well in the program.
- Decide where to allocate new resources.
- Document the level of success in accomplishing objectives.
- Demonstrate that accountability requirements are fulfilled.
- Aggregate information from several evaluations to estimate outcome effects for similar kinds of programs.
- Gather success stories. (CDC, 1999)

Affect Participants

- Reinforce intervention messages.
- Stimulate dialogue and raise awareness regarding health issues.
- Broaden consensus among coalition members regarding program goals.
- Teach evaluation skills to staff and other stakeholders.
- Support organizational change and development. (CDC, 1999)

Example Activities

- Meeting with stakeholders to clarify the intent or purpose of the evaluation;
- Learning which persons are in a position to actually use the findings, then orienting the plan to meet their needs;
- Understanding how the evaluation results are to be used;
- Writing explicit evaluation questions to be answered;
- Describing practical methods for sampling, data collection, data analysis, interpretation, and judgment;
- Preparing a written protocol or agreement that summarizes the evaluation procedures, with clear roles and responsibilities for all stakeholders; and
- Revising parts or all of the evaluation plan when critical circumstances change. (CDC, 1999)

Selected sources of evidence for an evaluation:

Persons

- Clients, program participants, nonparticipants;
- Staff, program managers, administrators;
- General public;
- Key informants;
- Funding officials;
- Critics/skeptics;
- Staff of other agencies;
- Representatives of advocacy groups;
- Elected officials, legislators, policymakers; and

- Local and state health officials. (CDC, 1999)

Documents

- Grant proposals, newsletters, press releases;
- Meeting minutes, administrative records, registration/enrollment forms;
- Publicity materials, quarterly reports;
- Publications, journal articles, posters;
- Previous evaluation reports;
- Asset and needs assessments;
- Surveillance summaries;
- Database records;
- Records held by funding officials or collaborators;
- Internet pages; and
- Graphs, maps, charts, photographs, videotapes. (CDC, 1999)

Observations

- Meetings, special events/activities, job performance; and
- Service encounters. (CDC, 1999)

Selected techniques for gathering evidence:

- Written survey (e.g. handout, telephone, fax, mail, e-mail, or Internet);
- Personal interview (e.g. individual or group; structured, semistructured, or conversational);
- Observation;
- Document analysis;
- Case study;

- Group assessment (e.g. brainstorming or nominal group [i.e., a structured group process conducted to elicit and rank priorities, set goals, or identify problems]);
- Role play, dramatization;
- Expert or peer review;
- Portfolio review;
- Testimonials;
- Semantic differentials, paired comparisons, similarity or dissimilarity tests;
- Hypothetical scenarios;
- Storytelling;
- Geographical mapping;
- Concept mapping;
- Pile sorting (i.e., a technique that allows respondents to freely categorize items, revealing how hey perceive the structure of a domain);
- Free-listing (i.e., a technique to elicit a complete list of all items in a cultural domain);
- Social network diagraming;
- Simulation, modeling;
- Debriefing sessions;
- Cost accounting;
- Photography, drawing, art, videography;
- Diaries or journals; and
- Logs, activity forms, registries. (CDC, 1999)

Gathering Credible Evidence

Example Activities

- Choosing indicators that meaningfully address evaluation questions;

- Describing fully the attributes of information sources and the rationale for their selection;
- Establishing clear procedures and training staff to collect high-quality information;
- Monitoring periodically the quality of information obtained and taking practical steps to improve quality;
- Estimating in advance the amount of information required or establishing criteria for deciding when to stop collecting data in situations where an iterative or evolving process is used; and
- Safeguarding the confidentiality of information and information sources. (CDC, 1999)

Selected sources of standards for judging program performance:

- Needs of participants;
- Community values, expectations, norms;
- Degree of participation;
- Program objectives;
- Program protocols and procedures;
- Expected performance, forecasts, estimates;
- Feasibility;
- Sustainability;
- Absence of harms;
- Targets or fixed criteria of performance;
- Change in performance over time;
- Performance by previous or similar programs;
- Performance by a control or comparison group;
- Resource efficiency;
- Professional standards;
- Mandates, policies, statutes, regulations, laws;

- Judgments by reference groups (e.g., participants, staff, experts, and funding officials);
- Institutional goals;
- Political ideology;
- Social equity;
- Political will; and
- Human rights. (CDC, 1999)

Justifying Conclusions

Example Activities

- Using appropriate methods of analysis and synthesis to summarize findings;
- Interpreting the significance of results for deciding what the findings mean;
- Making judgments according to clearly stated values that classify a result (e.g., as positive or negative and high or low);
- Considering alternative ways to compare results (e.g., compared with program objectives, a comparison group, national norms, past performance, or needs);
- Generating alternative explanations for findings and indicating why these explanations should or should not be discounted;
- Recommending actions or decisions that are consistent with the conclusions; and
- Limiting conclusions to situations, time periods, persons, contexts, and purposes for which the findings are applicable. (CDC, 1999)

Checklist for ensuring effective evaluation reports:

- Provide interim and final reports to intended users in time for use.
- Tailor the report content, format, and style for the audience(s) by involving audience members.
- Include a summary.
- Summarize the description of the stakeholders and how they were engaged.
- Describe essential features of the program (e.g., including logic models).
- Explain the focus of the evaluation and its limitations.
- Include an adequate summary of the evaluation plan and procedures.
- Provide all necessary technical information (e.g., in appendices).
- Specify the standards and criteria for evaluative judgments.
- Explain the evaluative judgments and how they are supported by the evidence.
- List both strengths and weaknesses of the evaluation.
- Discuss recommendations for action with their advantages, disadvantages, and resource implications.
- Ensure protections for program clients and other stakeholders.
- Anticipate how people or organizations might be affected by the findings.
- Present minority opinions or rejoinders where necessary.
- Verify that the report is accurate and unbiased.

- Organize the report logically and include appropriate details.
- Remove technical jargon.
- Use examples, illustrations, graphics, and stories. (CDC, 1999)

Ensuring use and sharing lessons learned:

Example Activities

- Designing the evaluation to achieve intended use by intended users;
- Preparing stakeholders for eventual use by rehearsing throughout the project how different kinds of conclusions would affect program operations;
- Providing continuous feedback to stakeholders regarding interim findings, provisional interpretations, and decisions to be made that might affect likelihood of use;
- Scheduling follow-up meetings with intended users to facilitate the transfer of evaluation conclusions into appropriate actions or decisions; and
- Disseminating both the procedures used and the lessons learned from the evaluation to stakeholders, using tailored communications strategies that meet their particular needs. (CDC, 1999)

Utility Standards

The following utility standards ensure that an evaluation will serve the information needs of intended users:

A. **Stakeholder identification.** Persons involved in or affected by the evaluation should be identified so that their needs can be addressed.
B. **Evaluator credibility.** The persons conducting the evaluation should be trustworthy and competent in performing the evaluation for findings to achieve maximum credibility and acceptance.
C. **Information scope and selection.** Information collected should address pertinent questions regarding the program and be responsive to the needs and interests of clients and other specified stakeholders.
D. **Values identification.** The perspectives, procedures, and rationale used to interpret the findings should be carefully described so that the bases for value judgments are clear.
E. **Report clarity.** Evaluation reports should clearly describe the program being evaluated, including its context and the purposes, procedures, and findings of the evaluation so that essential information is provided and easily understood.
F. **Report timeliness and dissemination.** Substantial interim findings and evaluation reports should be disseminated to intended users so that they can be used in a timely fashion.
G. **Evaluation impact.** Evaluations should be planned, conducted, and reported in ways that

encourage follow-through by stakeholders to increase the likelihood of the evaluation being used. (CDC, 1999)

Feasibility Standards

The following feasibility standards ensure that an evaluation will be realistic, prudent, diplomatic, and frugal:

A. **Practical procedures.** Evaluation procedures should be practical while needed information is being obtained to keep disruption to a minimum.
B. **Political viability.** During planning and conduct of the evaluation, consideration should be given to the varied positions of interest groups so that their cooperation can be obtained and possible attempts by any group to curtail evaluation operations or to bias or misapply the results can be averted or counteracted.
C. **Cost-effectiveness.** The evaluation should be efficient and produce valuable information to justify expended resources. (CDC, 1999)

Propriety Standards

The following propriety standards ensure that an evaluation will be conducted legally, ethically, and with regard for the welfare of those involved in the evaluation as well as those affected by its results:

A. **Service orientation.** The evaluation should be designed to assist organizations in addressing and

serving effectively the needs of the targeted participants.
B. **Formal agreements.** All principal parties involved in an evaluation should agree in writing to their obligations (i.e., what is to be done, how, by whom, and when) so that each must adhere to the conditions of the agreement or renegotiate it.
C. **Rights of human subjects.** The evaluation should be designed and conducted in a manner that respects and protects the rights and welfare of human subjects.
D. **Human interactions.** Evaluators should interact respectfully with other persons associated with an evaluation, so that participants are not threatened or harmed.
E. **Complete and fair assessment.** The evaluation should be complete and fair in its examination and recording of strengths and weaknesses of the program so that strengths can be enhanced and problem areas addressed.
F. **Disclosure of findings.** The principal parties to an evaluation should ensure that the full evaluation findings with pertinent limitations are made accessible to the persons affected by the evaluation and any others with expressed legal rights to receive the results.
G. **Conflict of interest.** Conflict of interest should be handled openly and honestly so that the evaluation processes and results are not compromised.
H. **Fiscal responsibility.** The evaluator's allocation and expenditure of resources should reflect sound accountability procedures by being prudent and

ethically responsible, so that expenditures are accountable and appropriate. (CDC, 1999)

Accuracy Standards

The following accuracy standards ensure that an evaluation will convey technically adequate information regarding the determining features of merit of the program:

A. **Program documentation.** The program being evaluated should be documented clearly and accurately.
B. **Context analysis.** The context in which the program exists should be examined in enough detail to identify probable influences on the program.
C. **Described purposes and procedures.** The purposes and procedures of the evaluation should be monitored and described in enough detail to identify and assess them.
D. **Defensible information sources.** Sources of information used in a program evaluation should be described in enough detail to assess the adequacy of the information.
E. **Valid information.** Information-gathering procedures should be developed and implemented to ensure a valid interpretation for the intended use.
F. **Reliable information.** Information-gathering procedures should be developed and implemented to ensure sufficiently reliable information for the intended use.

G. **Systematic information.** Information collected, processed, and reported in an evaluation should be systematically reviewed and any errors corrected.
H. **Analysis of quantitative information.** Quantitative information should be analyzed appropriately and systematically so that evaluation questions are answered effectively.
I. **Analysis of qualitative information.** Qualitative information should be analyzed appropriately and systematically to answer evaluation questions effectively.
J. **Justified conclusions.** Conclusions reached should be explicitly justified for stakeholders' assessment.
K. **Impartial reporting.** Reporting procedures should guard against the distortion caused by personal feelings and biases of any party involved in the evaluation to reflect the findings fairly.
L. **Metaevaluation.** The evaluation should be formatively and summatively evaluated against these and other pertinent standards to guide its conduct appropriately and, on completion, to enable close examination of its strengths and weaknesses by stakeholders. (CDC, 1999)

Logic Modeling in Program Evaluation

Example Format for a Logic Model

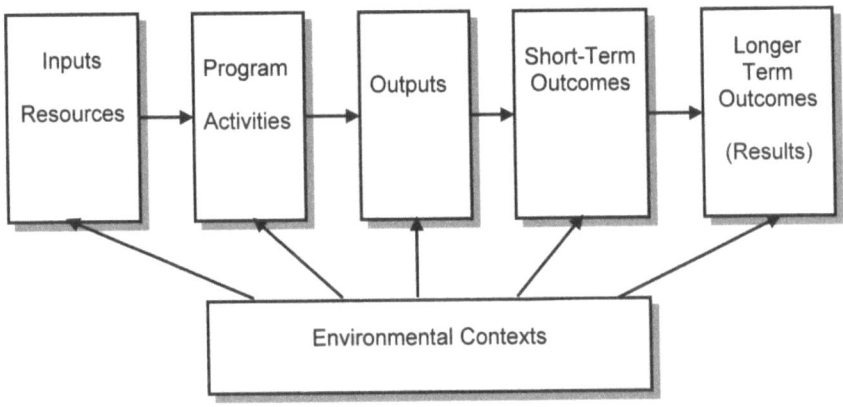

Once a need is established for a health program, goals and outcomes related directly to the need must be written. Goals and outcomes should be strong and measurable because they establish focus for the program and the basis for assessment and evaluation. They should also align to criteria established by stakeholders or standards.

Let's take a look at various evaluation frameworks, designs, or models. The chosen framework represents the way the components to be evaluated are arranged, observed, or manipulated to answer your original evaluation question.

According to Kellogg (2004), a logic model is a systemic and visual way "to present and share your understanding of the relationships among the resources you have to operate your program, the activities you plan, and the changes or results you hope to achieve." The logic model uses words and/or pictures to describe activities thought to bring about the needed changes to result in your desired outcome. Logic models are used by program planners and evaluators to identify program inputs, activities, outputs, and outcomes.

Typically, outcomes are classified as immediate, intermediate, long-term, and ultimate. Evaluators can use logic models to lead program staff in discussions about how their program might achieve its goals and objectives and the program elements to be evaluated at a certain time.

Theory-driven evaluation involves developing a theory for why a program should achieve its desired outcomes. Because development of a program theory requires broad stakeholder commitment, it increases the likelihood that all program elements will receive appropriate attention and that evaluation activities will lead to program improvement. A program theory serves as the foundation for development of evaluation questions and decisions on what to study and when to collect data. A theory-driven approach is useful in program planning in addition to evaluation of existing programs.

Decision-oriented models also are frequently used in healthcare. The CIPP Model (Context, Input, Process, and Product) is quite popular in educational settings. Context evaluation is getting the big picture of the program. Here is where you will decide how and where the program and evaluation fit. The target population is identified, and assessment of its needs is completed. Input evaluation includes information collection related to the mission, goals, and plans of the program. Strategies for meeting the outcomes or goals are addressed at this stage. Process evaluation analyzes the quality of the program implementation. The evaluator will use these data to modify the project to improve the overall outcomes of the project or program. Finally, the product evaluation is where the positives and negatives of the program are reviewed. The effects of the program on the participants are also addressed. Measurements of the strengths and weaknesses of the program are identified to support the improvement of upcoming programs.

Decision-Oriented Approach or the CIPP Model

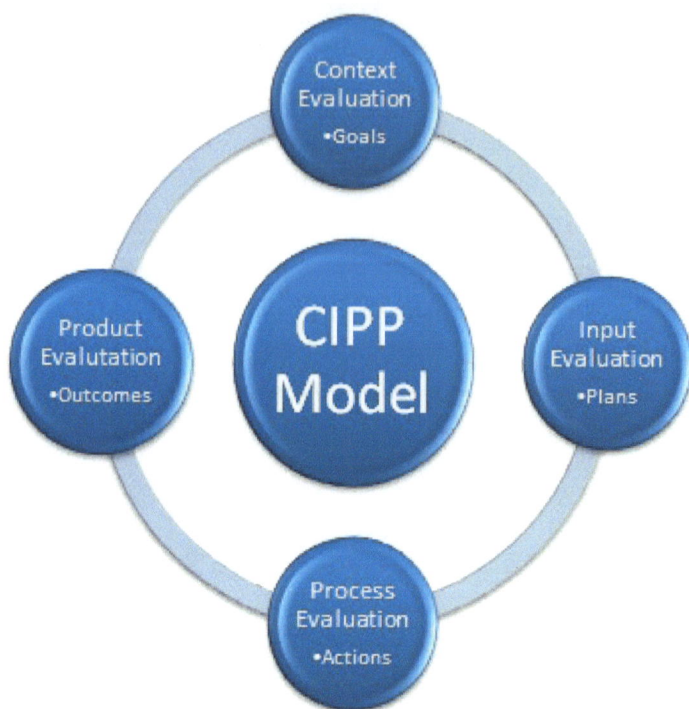

The design of the program evaluation might use the **Decision-Oriented Approach or the CIPP Model** which includes the following categories:

- Context – Get the big picture.
- Input – Collect information.
- Process – Analyze implementation quality.
- Product – Review the program's positives and negatives.

A logic model is a planning and evaluation tool. Logic models are used to plan, describe, manage, communicate, and evaluate an intervention or program. A model is an abstraction designed to identify important elements and relationships within a system. An evaluation logic model tool is used to understand relationships between program activities, its consequences, and its environment (Morell, 2010).

Usually a picture that addresses any or all of three questions:

- If a program works as intended, what will be different? (Summative evaluation)
- What does it take for a program to work as intended? (Formative evaluation)
- What is needed to sustain a program after start-up? (Sustainability evaluation). (Morell, 2010)

In addition, logic models can:

- Represents views (consensus?) of some (all?) stakeholders.
- Work in progress, evolves with program, evaluation findings. (Morell, 2010)

A logic model can be effective in program evaluation and increase the likelihood that program efforts will be successful and includes the following components:

- Communicate the purpose of the program and expected results.
- Describe the actions expected to lead to the desired results.
- Become a reference point for everyone involved in the program.

- Improve program staff expertise in planning, implementation, and evaluation.
- Involve stakeholders, enhancing the likelihood of resource commitment.
- Incorporate findings from other research and demonstration projects.
- Identify potential obstacles to program operation so that staff can address them early on. (CDC, 2017).

The benefits of logic modeling can help evaluate a state program as a whole and offer a more detailed view of any specific intervention or component of a program, such as developing a state plan or a health communication campaign (CDC, 2017).

Drawbacks of Logic Modeling

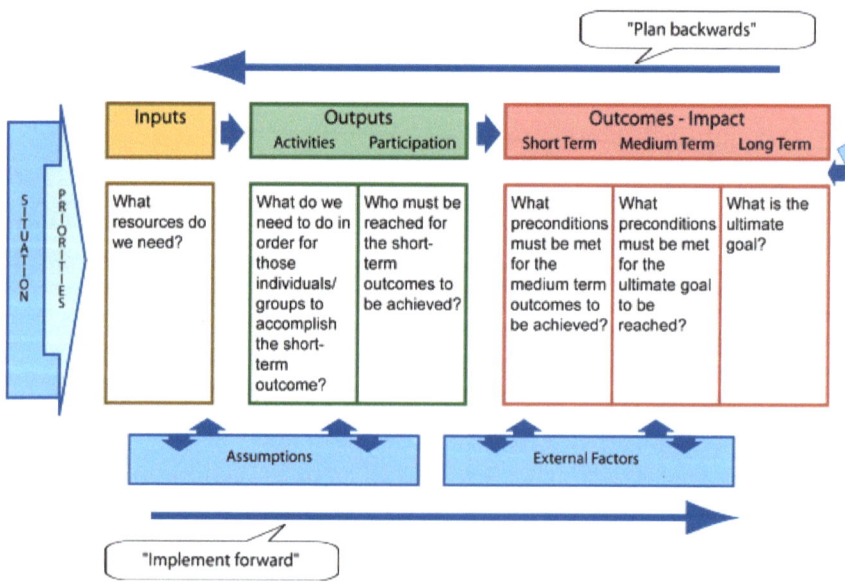

Incompleteness & error: The system behavior view:

- Because a deterministic model cannot fully specify an open system, logic models are always incomplete approximations.
- Model stability often depends on a careful balance among several factors. Small perturbation in any one can causer major change in the system.
- Error potential increases with:
  - Length of causal chains
  - Number of feedback loops
  - Network richness (nodes:edges)
  - Accuracy of assumptions (e.g., does an element really belong in the model? Is there really a feedback loop? Does "A" really cause "B"?)
  - Program's departure from previous solutions
    - Small change + proven program + known setting vs.
    - Innovative program + innovative solution + novel setting
    - Rate of change in program or its environment. (Morell, 2010)

Incompleteness and error: The domain expertise view:

- Reasonable people may think of program theory by drawing on different experience and bodies of research.
- Can we really say who is right?
- Is there much likelihood that any of them will get it completely right?

- Do we really think all these people will have the same program theory, thus driving the same methodologies and metrics? (Morell, 2010)

SMART Goals

S.M.A.R.T. Goals Defined

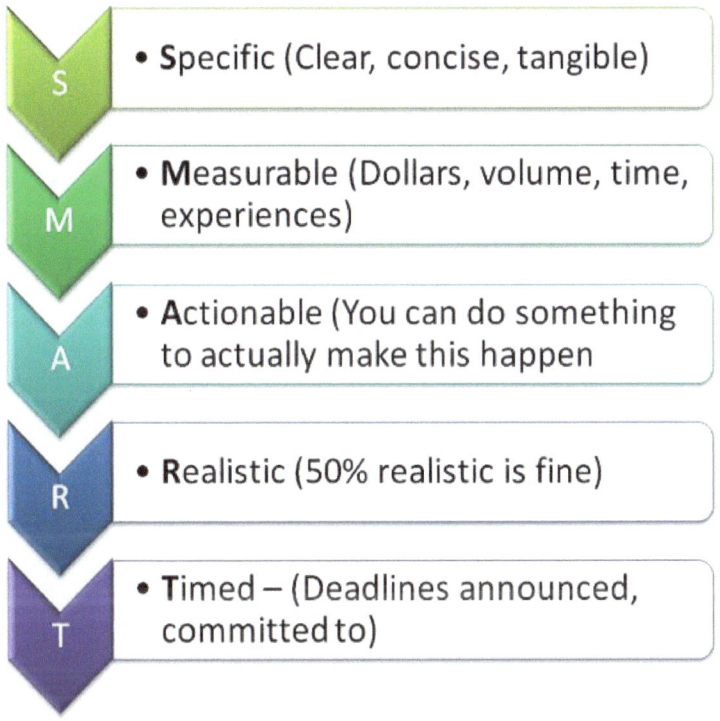

- **S**pecific (Clear, concise, tangible)
- **M**easurable (Dollars, volume, time, experiences)
- **A**ctionable (You can do something to actually make this happen
- **R**ealistic (50% realistic is fine)
- **T**imed – (Deadlines announced, committed to)

The concept of SMART goals was posited by George T. Doran in 1981 who was a former director and consultant of corporate planning for Washington Water Power Company. He published a paper called, "There's a S.M.A.R.T. Way to Write Management's Goals and Objectives." Doran recommended S.M.A.R.T. goals as a mechanism or means to develop a benchmark to assist and enhance the accomplishment of goals (Esposito, 2015; University of Virginia: Employee Development, n.d.).

Specific
Measurable
Achievable
Relevant
Time-Bound

A study conducted by Tregoning (2014) revealed steps that can be taken in any workplace environment or when evaluating the effectiveness of a health care system or program.

5 Step Linear Approach to Risk Assessment

1. Getting started. What are you trying to achieve? Who needs to be involved?
2. Identifying health priorities. Gathering data.
3. Assessing a health priority for action. Determining effective actions.
4. Planning for change. Clarifying intervention aims. Action planning.
5. Moving on/review. Measuring impact. Choosing the next priority. (Tregoning, 2014)

5 Steps to Risk Assessment

1. Identify the hazards.
2. Decide who might be harmed and how.
3. Evaluate the risks and decide on precaution.
4. Record your findings and implement them.
5. Review your assessment and update if necessary. (Tregoning, 2014)

SMART goals for the program in the case study included the following:

1. Assess and measure employee access to self-refer to occupational health (OH) where they are able to access early intervention and treatment as appropriate.
2. Assess and measure access to health and wellbeing advice.
3. Assess and measure health interventions through the occupational health (OH) service.
4. Assess and measure access to physiotherapy, health advice, and stress counseling.
5. Assess and measure the aim of promoting health for all employees and as a tool for supporting a healthy workforce.
6. Assess and measure the promotion of health services through the health board intranet site, leaflets, posters, seminars for managers and employees, and from within the occupational health (OH) department.
7. Assess and measure the aim of this service through its dedicated intranet page providing easily accessible information and a resource for self-help and signposting for health promotion and other initiatives. (Tregoning, 2014)

One popular method of measuring plan performance is the audit. Audits are simply a formal review of the objectives and alignment of performance of the plan to the objectives. The key to a successful audit process is to identify the major functions of the plan and then determine key industry or internal measures of performance and satisfaction. An audit may also examine regulatory compliance or adherence to policies and procedures.

According to Pincus, Spaeth-Rublee and Watkins (2011), "Over the past decade, efforts to measure and improve quality have permeated health policy and health care generally but have barely penetrated mental health and substance abuse care" (p. 730).

Moreover, Pincus, Spaeth-Rublee and Watkins (2011) stated:
> In fact, not long after the National Committee for Quality Assurance reported that despite important gains in quality in the general medical/surgical sector, "there are…disturbing exceptions to this pattern of [overall health care quality] improvement. The quality of care for Americans with mental health problems remains as poor today as it was several years ago." (p. 730)

Approaches to Conducting an Audit

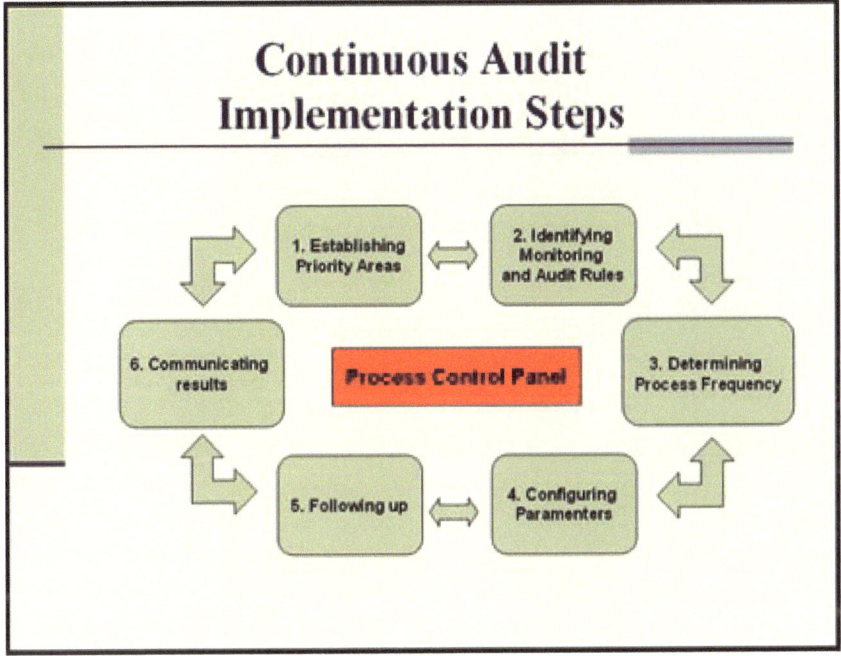

Might involve the following actions and considerations:

First, the plan to be reviewed must be selected. This could be an overall human resources plan for the institution, or it could be in the form of a specific plan individually.

Second, key performance measures would be identified as a benchmark for success. Some of the areas that may be measured are programs such as staffing, benefits, compensation, appraisals, and training and development plans.

Third step is to gather the appropriate data for analysis. Much of the data to be collected is found in organizational documents, but sometimes the human resources department needs to create other ways of collecting data. Many times, the use of technology databases and auditing software is appropriate.

The last step is to analyze the data collected from the audit. The human resources specialist will review the data to determine satisfaction levels, effectiveness, efficiencies, and the economic value. Ultimately, the analysis will produce a declaration of whether or not the audited program achieved the preset goals based on the measurement metrics.

Although many government agencies audit and get audited, those recommendations for improvement don't always take affect or end up helping the people they should be serving.

Pincus, Spaeth-Rublee, and Watkins (2011) noted that the Institute of Medicine committee's report on mental health care offered various recommendations that have basically been ignored by the mental health community and system.

> Remarkably, the response to these recommendations has been tepid, at best. No entity has stepped in to take responsibility for leadership in implementing these recommendations. There have been no announcements of major new initiatives or programs in this regard from federal agencies or major nongovernmental organizations.

No coordinated efforts for research programs to develop better methods or measures have emerged from major federal research agencies or foundations.

What's more, the National Committee for Quality Assurance's Healthcare Effectiveness Data and Information Set measures have not greatly improved, and fewer than 5 percent of the National Quality Forum's list of more than 650 vetted indicators specifically relate to care for people with mental health and substance use conditions. (Pincus, Spaeth-Rublee, & Watkins, 2011, 731)

Guiding Principles of Evaluation

Guiding principles of evaluation (part 1) includes the following:

1. Evaluation principles and purposes
    a. Important principles of evaluation are:
        1) Evaluators conduct systematic, data-based inquiries to:
            a) Ensure the accuracy and credibility of the evaluation information they produce
            b) Communicate their methods and approaches accurately and in sufficient detail to allow others to understand, interpret, critique, and apply their results
        2) Evaluators provide competent performance to stakeholders.

      a) Demonstrate cultural competence to ensure recognition, accurate interpretations, and respect for diversity
      b) Practice within the limits of professional training and competence
  3) Evaluators display honesty and integrity in their own behaviors and attempt to ensure the honesty and integrity of the evaluation process.
  4) Evaluators respect the security, dignity, and self-worth of respondents, program participants, clients, and other evaluation stakeholders.
  5) Evaluators articulate and take into account the diversity of general and public interests and values that may relate to the evaluation.

Guiding principles of evaluation (part 2) includes the following:

  b. Purposes of evaluation in training
    1) General purposes of evaluation include:
      a) Improving products, personnel, programs, organizations, governments, consumers, and public interest
      b) Contributing to informed decision making and an enlightened change
      c) Empowering stakeholders by collecting data from them and engaging them in the evaluation process
      d) Providing new insights
      e) Constructing and providing the best possible information concerning the value of whatever is being evaluated

Guiding principles of evaluation (part 3) includes the following:

2) Other purposes
   a) One purpose of evaluation in training is to provide results to the appropriate stakeholders
   b) Another purpose of evaluation in training is to make decisions regarding:
      (1) Efficiency: the degree to which a program or project has been productive in relationship to its resources. Questions to answer regarding a program's efficiency include:
         (a) When did the program or project begin?
         (b) Did the program or project result in an improvement? What kind or kinds of improvement or improvements?
         (c) How long did it take to achieve the results?
      (2) Effectiveness: the degree to which the goals of the program or project have been reached. Questions to answer regarding a program's effectiveness include:
         (a) What did the program do?
         (b) How well did the program do it?
         (c) What were the outcomes of the program?
      (3) Effect: the degree to which the program or project resulted in change. Questions to answer regarding a program's efficiency include:

(a) Did the program influence lives?
(b) Did the program improve a situation or resolve an issue?

Reasons to evaluate include the following:

c) Funding purposes, for example state or federally funded programs
d) Comparison purposes. Which of several methods is most effective?
e) Make the case for a new program
f) Justify a current program or a project
   (1) Did you accomplish what you set out to do?
   (2) How does the program compare to similar efforts?
g) Improve or change a program
3) To determine the eventual use of evaluation data and who might make use of the results; Kirkpatrick (1994) has identified four levels of evaluation:
   a) Level one: participant impressions
   b) Level two: effectiveness of the program
   c) Level three: effect on the participants
   d) Level four: return on investment for the organization

When considering decision making related to evaluation, it is important to keep in mind the following principles:

4) Everyone involved in the program, from those who fund it, to those who lead it, to those who

receive its services or products, has a stake in the decision making.
5) Monitoring provides information that may be used to aid in decisions about improving, continuing, or discontinuing a program.

Decision making must be based on evaluating each phase of the program planning cycle as shown below:

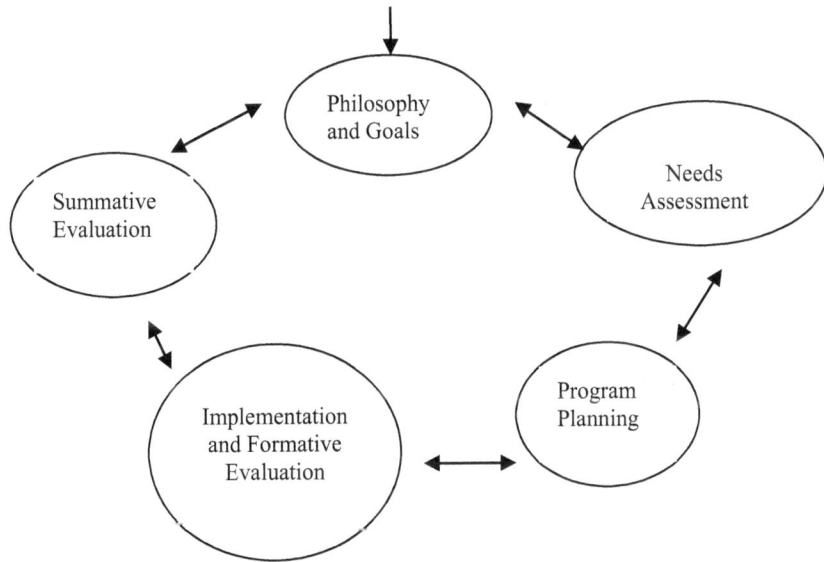

The Evaluator's Role

a) The evaluator's role in the philosophy and goals phase is to help identify the connection between program goals and the client's needs that must be addressed.
b) The evaluator's role in the needs assessment phase is to assist in identifying the needs, to make the link between what the program sees as its mission or goals and those

identified needs, and to look at the effectiveness of previous program activities compared to the mission.

c) The evaluator's role in the program planning phase is to help program planners to develop, adapt, or select an evaluation design to meet their needs.

d) The evaluator's role in the program implementation and formative evaluation phase is to look at the client's progress toward attaining goals and the staff's effectiveness in performing activities.

e) The evaluator's role in the summative evaluation phase is to document program processes and to measure the attainment of specified goals.

Effective Evaluation Models

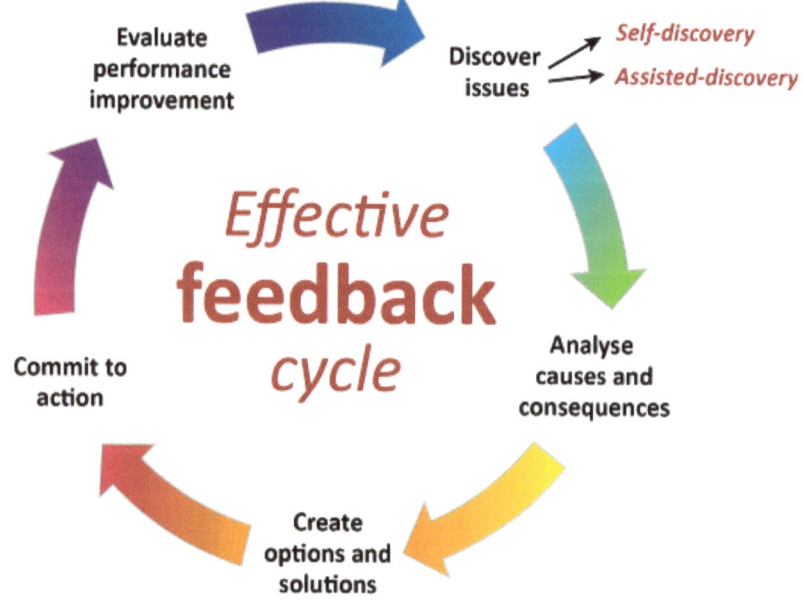

Effective evaluation models (part 1) include the following:

6) Discrepancy model
   a) This model is used when there is an understanding that a program does not exist in a vacuum, but instead exists within a complex organizational structure.
   b) In this model, there is more interest in why something occurred than in the fact that it did occur.
   c) When using this model, a program's developmental stages are examined with an understanding that each of the stages has a set of standards of performance.
   d) This model helps one to make decisions based on the difference between preset standards and what actually exists at each stage.
7) Goal-free model
   a) This evaluation model looks at a program's actual effect on identified needs.
   b) This model examines what the program is doing and how it addresses the needs in the client population.
   c) Program goals are not the criteria on which this evaluation model is based.
8) Transaction model
   a) It combines monitoring with process evaluation through a continuous interaction between the evaluator and the program or project staff.

b) The evaluator is an active participant, providing constant feedback.
c) The evaluator uses a variety of observational and interview techniques to obtain information from program staff and clients.

Effective evaluation models (part 2) include the following:

9) Decision making model
    a) Used to make decisions regarding future use of the program
    b) Concerned with long-range effects, rather than current performance
    c) Quantitative and qualitative methods might be employed in this model.
10) Goal-based model
    a) Only concerned with stated goals or objectives
    b) The evaluator looks to measure specified outcome variables, using quantitative or qualitative methods, including control or comparison groups.
11) Determining which model to use depends on the answer to the question "Why evaluate this program?"
    a) Is the program being evaluated to determine whether and to what degree the objectives of the program have been or are being achieved?
    b) Is the program being evaluated to make a decision regarding the future of the program?

Ethics Self-Assessment

Of what value is an ethics self-assessment?

The purpose and rationale for an ethics self-assessment is to abide by a code of ethics which might include a standard of conduct, ethical behavior, and a guide for healthcare practitioners in professional settings. An individual or a system, such as practitioners and the entire USA Health System, can assess their ethical standards when working in leadership roles as well as the actions they take with others based on a code of ethics. An ethical code of standards can assist in identifying areas with strong or weak ethical grounds. (ACHE, 2017)

Question to ask:

1. Who creates the code of ethics?
2. What standards are being used?
3. What ethics are considered?
4. What framework, model, or philosophy is present?
5. Who created the framework, model, or philosophy?
6. What is the agenda?

Cognitive Dissonance

Naturally, individuals can reject facts as facts can offend or damage their wrongly and strongly held beliefs. When one's worldview is changed by the infusion of new information, individuals may either reject the new information or change their beliefs and incorporate the new knowledge.

Portugal (2015) stated:

> Strengths and weaknesses of transformative learning theory can be either a positive transformation in the learners' thinking or a cognitive dissonance. When transformative learning techniques are applied in a learning environment, the learner has the choice of either changing his or her previous ways of thinking and adopting a new way of viewing his or her world, or the learner can decide to reject the new information, and cognitive dissonance may be the result (McFalls & Cobb-Roberts, 2001). When learners experience social and cultural change that does not fit into their schema or worldview, the result can be a transformation or cognitive dissonance. The concept of cognitive dissonance theory applies to individuals who are not cognitively ready for new information and who may reject this information as it creates discord with their previously held beliefs (McFalls & Cobb-Roberts, 2001). A discord of cognition requires that one either transforms his or her way of thinking, being, or doing, or is forced to rationalize or justify his or her beliefs, attitudes, and behaviors (McFalls & Cobb-Roberts, 2001). Cognitive dissonance is the result of receiving new information that challenges one's old and firmly held beliefs, which are in opposition or contrary to the new information (J. Green, 1998). (p. 31)

PURPOSE & LOGIC MODEL

The purpose identified for this evaluation is to assess the quality and ability of a health system or health education program to provide services, education, healing treatments, and remedies to affected populations in the country. Systems, treatments, and education programs can be discussed and examined for effectiveness and failure. The following graphical depiction or logic model provides information on inputs, activities, outputs, and outcomes (CDC, 2017; SAMHSA, 2015; SAMHSA; 2016)

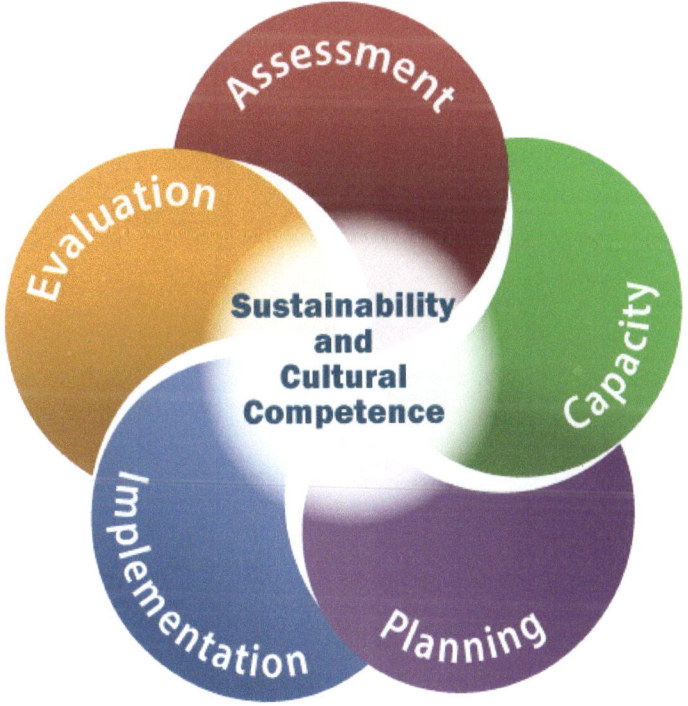

(SAMHSA, 2015)

Outcomes-based Logic Model

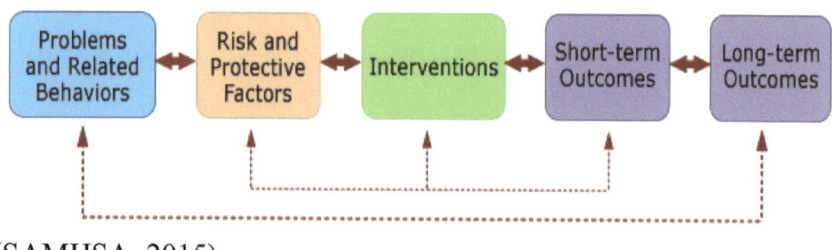

(SAMHSA, 2015)

More Components in Program Evaluation

Thinking Through a Logic Model
   Resources/Inputs
   - What resources are available to support the program being evaluated (e.g., staff, money, space, time, partnerships, technology, etc.)?

   Activities
   - What specific activities are undertaken (or planned) to achieve the outcomes?

   Outputs
   - What products (e.g., materials, units of services delivered) are produced by your staff as a result of the activities performed?

   Outcomes
   - What are the program's intended outcomes (intended outcomes are short-term, intermediate, or long-term)?
   - What do you ultimately want to change as a result of your activities (long-term outcomes)?
   - What occurs between your activities and the point at which you see these ultimate outcomes (short-term and intermediate outcomes)?

Proposed Timeline
- In what timeframe will the evaluation occur?
- When will significant events, such as formal data collection, data analysis, information dissemination, take place?
- Are there any foreseeable bottlenecks or sequencing issues?

Potential Evaluation Budget
- What is the estimated cost for this evaluation?
- Where will the monetary and other resources originate to support the evaluation?

What are Inputs, Outputs, Outcomes and Impact?

The Logic Model Approach

INPUTS → **ACTIVITIES** → **OUTPUTS** → **OUTCOMES** → **IMPACT**

- Resources dedicated to or consumed by the project
- Usually a NOUN staff, facilities, money, time…

- What the project does with inputs to fulfill its mission
- Usually a GERUND a verb in its "-ing" form, such as assessing, enabling, reviewing…

- The volume of work accomplished by the project
- Usually a QUANTITY the number of projects, the number of case studies…

- Benefits or changes for participants during or after project activities
- Usually a CHANGE better projects, increased skills…

- The long term consequences of the intervention
- A fundamental CHANGE intended or unintended in a system or society

Your Planned Work | **Your Intended Results**

Program Action – Logic Model

Situation
Needs & assets
Symptoms v problems
Stakeholder engagement

Priorities
CONSIDER
Mission
Vision
Values
Mandates
Resources
Local dynamics
Collaborators
Competitors
INTENDED OUTCOMES

INPUT	OUTPUT		OUTCOMES/IMPACT		
Investments	Activities	Participants	Short-term	Medium-term	Long-term
Staff Volunteers Time Money Research base Materials Equipment Technology Partners	Conduct workshops, meetings Deliver services Develop products, curriculum, resources Train Provide counseling Assess Facilitate Partner Work with media	Clients Agencies Decision makers Customers Satisfaction	Learning: Awareness Knowledge Attitudes Skill Opinions Aspirations Motivations	Action: Behavior Practice Decision making Policies Social action	Conditions: Social Economic Civic Environmental

Assumptions   External Factors

EVALUATION
FOCUS • COLLECT DATA • ANALYZE & INTERPRET • REPORT

Program Action – Logic Model

Situation
- Needs and assets
- Symptoms versus problems
- Stakeholder engagement

Priorities
Consider:
- Mission
- Vision
- Values
- Mandates
- Resources
- Local Dynamics
- Collaborators
- Competitors

Intended Outcomes

Inputs

What we invest
- Staff
- Volunteers
- Time
- Money
- Research base
- Materials
- Equipment
- Technology
- Partners

Outputs

Activities

What we do
- Conduct workshops, meetings
- Deliver services
- Develop products, curriculum, resources
- Train
- Provide counseling
- Assess
- Facilitate
- Partner
- Work with media

Participation

Who we reach
- Participants
- Clients
- Agencies
- Decision-makers
- Customers

Outcomes – Impact

Short Term
What the short term results are
- Learning
- Awareness
- Knowledge
- Attitudes
- Skills
- Opinions
- Aspirations
- Motivations

Medium Term
What the medium term results are
- Action
- Behavior
- Practice
- Decision-making
- Policies
- Social Action

Long Term
What the ultimate impact(s) is
- Conditions
- Social
- Economic
- Civic
- Environmental

Assumptions   External Factors

Evaluation
Focus – Collect Data – Analyze and Interpret – Report

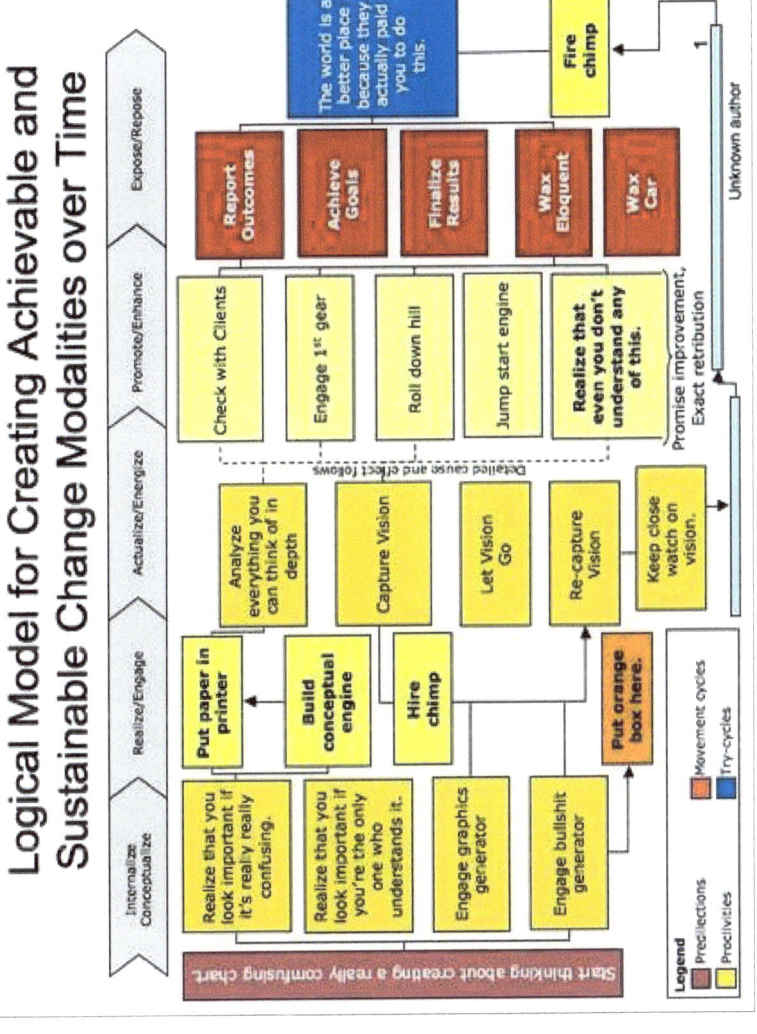

RESOURCES (INPUTS)	ACTIVITIES (PROCESSES)	RESULTS (OUTPUTS OR OUTCOMES)
People Infrastructure Materials (i.e. vaccine) Information Technology	1. What is done 2. How it is done	Health services delivered Change in health behavior Change in health status Patient Satisfaction

EVALUATION DESIGN

A simple input-output model:

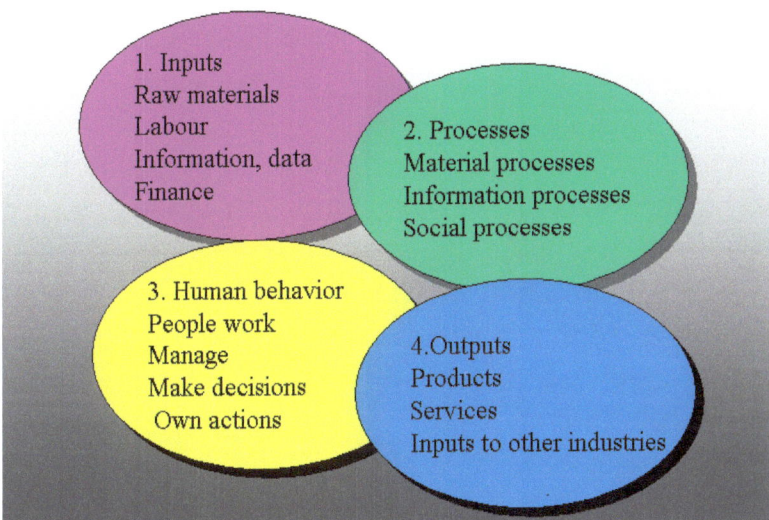

The evaluation design choice reflects the questions that need to be addressed and directs the scope and purpose of this process. The ultimate goal is to evaluate whether a system or program meets and serves the needs of individuals, how well they are served, and what the affects of that service has had in the lives of those individuals, families, and the communities. Stakeholder information needs emerging from the evaluation provide a basis for: (1) which treatments have failed and why, (2) what types of information needs to be disseminated to better inform the public, and (3) how to better serve the affected.

Evaluation Design

The design of a program evaluation might use the **Decision-Oriented Approach or the CIPP Model** which includes the following categories:

- Context – Get the big picture.
- Input – Collect information.
- Process – Analyze implementation quality.
- Product – Review the program's positives and negatives.

The selection of this design was chosen because of the broad nature and scope of the evaluation. A "big picture" view of a system including strategies, methods, techniques, treatments, management, and philosophy is necessary to address systemic problems. Information can be easily collected via published research, longitudinal statistics, the Internet, and interviews. The analysis of program quality is addressed along with the positives and negatives encountered by those served by the system.
The **Outcomes-Based Logic Model** was chosen for this evaluation because it fits well with the purpose and scope of the evaluation design. The purpose is to evaluate if the treatments and/or education model used by the system are effective.

Overall Evaluation Goals

The evaluation of processes and outcomes is the focus of this project and the following questions are asked:
1. How can the program be revised to better serve stakeholders?
2. Is the program sufficiently meeting its intended need?
3. Should funding be continued?

SMART Measurable goals and outcomes include the following:

Specific
Measurable
Achievable
Relevant
Time-Bound (Esposito, 2015; University of Virginia: Employee Development, n.d.)

- What have been the negative consequences on individuals served by the system or program?
- How has the system or program met and served the needs of the affected populations?
- What evidence is present that reveals success or failure?
- How can individuals be better served; where and who can better serve individuals in need?

DATA COLLECTION
Program Evaluation Components

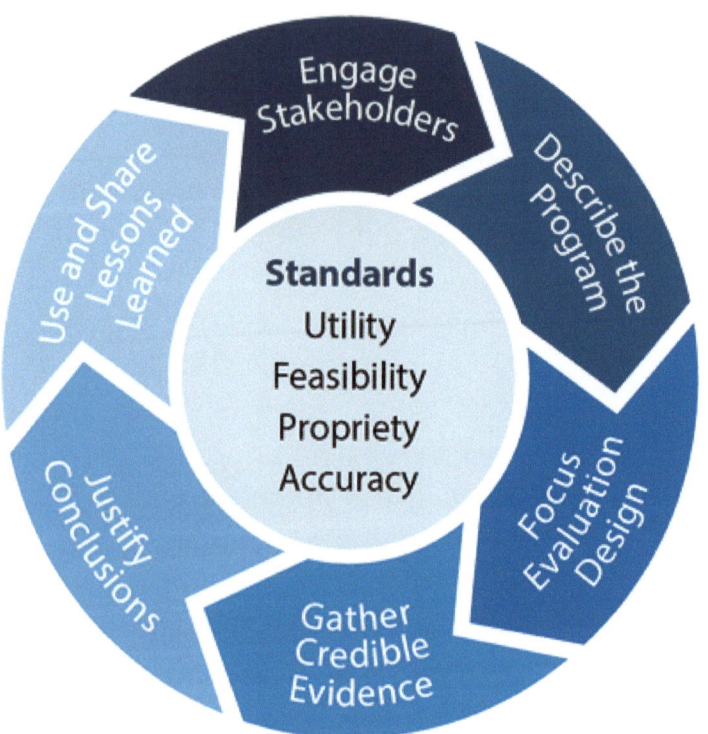

A program evaluation is a technical report that consists of various and specific components. According to the literature adapted from McNamara (2007), Survedi and Morford (2003), and Wilde and Sockey (1995), a program evaluation contains the following components that are sequenced in order: (1) title page, (2) executive summary which includes guiding questions, evaluation methods, key findings, conclusion, and key recommendations, (3) introduction and background which includes purpose of the program or project, purpose and aim of the evaluation, guiding evaluation questions, goals and objectives of the evaluation, evaluator relationship to the program, and rationale for selection of the program, (4) evaluation methodology which includes research design, sample and setting, data collection, measurement methods, data analysis, protection of human rights, limits of design, and best practices, (5) findings which includes hard and soft data, (6) summary discussion, (7) recommendations, (8) references, and (9) appendices. Some common types of program evaluations are the following: (1) outcomes-based, (2) goals-based, and (3) process-based (McNamara, 2007). According to Fitzpatrick, Sanders, and Worthen (2004), five different approaches to program evaluation include: (1) objective-oriented, (2) management-oriented, (3) consumer-oriented, (4) expertise-oriented, and (5) participant-oriented.

Quantitative & Qualitative Research Approaches
Compare & Contrast

Qualitative	Quantitative
Like Easy Awkward Slow Squirrel Efficient Ambiguous How Confusing	23,406 4.3 2m32s 76.8% $45,849 1,127 3.76% €12.75

Qualitative data are nonnumeric and this type of data takes the form of verbal descriptions and narrative. Quantitative data is numerical in form and statistics are oftentimes used to summarize the data. According to Onwuegbuzie and Leech (2007), typically only one type of statistical generalization is relevant in quantitative research, which specifically relates to "generalizing findings from the sample to the underlying population" (p. 240). These researchers posited three types of generalizations which include case-to-case, analytic, and statistical. Quantitative surveys lend well to circumstances where groups being researched are larger while qualitative surveys are better suited when groups are smaller or somewhat marginalized and where there might be more difficulty administering a survey. This approach to data collection may provide more detail, context, outreach, analysis, and a richer interpretation of the data depending upon one's program evaluation. These methods of data collection may be considered more empirically sound and can be reproduced more reliably.

According to the literature, quantitative researchers have believed that this method corrects the weaknesses of qualitative research. Young (2007) stated that traditional qualitative research tends "to be anecdotal, noncomparative, atheoretical, too legalistic, too descriptive, and not falsifiable" (p. 4). In addition, Young (2007) posited that quantitative research is "generalizeable, comparable, theory-based, explanatory, and falisifiable" (p. 4). Quantitative data is represented in numerical form while qualitative data is represented in text or narrative form. In addition, methods used to collect data can be quantitative such as large, representative surveys while qualitative research includes data collection methods such as observations and interviews (Rao & Woolcock, 2003, p. 169).

Table 2
Compare & Contrast Quantitative & Qualitative Methods

Quantitative Research	*Qualitative Research*
numeric data is simple	data is rich or complex
Measurement	Meaning
Explanation	Understanding
Prediction	Interpretation
Generalized explanation	Contextual explanation
population sample is representative	sample is purposive and a representative perspective
Hypothesis-testing	Exploratory
Claims objectivity	Accepts subjectivity
experimental control closed system	ecological validity open system

From "Qualitative Inquiry and Research Design: Choosing Among Five Traditions," by J. W. Creswell, 1998.

Having the ability to make generalizations

Quantitative approaches to program evaluation are viewed by researchers as having the ability to make generalizations about large populations based upon smaller representative samples of the population. Quantitative approaches can help authenticate and verify "the impact of given variables on project outcomes" when presented with a set of identifiable traits or characteristics (Rao & Woolcock, 2003, p. 166). Furthermore, other researchers can copy, repeat, or duplicate the study and thus validate the original findings. When incorporating quantitative methods in program evaluation, the researcher is removed from the individuals being studied. Data collection and analysis is in numerical form and quantitative methods are viewed by researchers as empirically rigorous, objective, impartial, and maintaining sound research standards.

Unlike quantitative methods, when qualitative methods to program evaluation are used, the researcher may be intimately involved in the data collection. Data collection and analysis is in interview and narrative form. Qualitative methods to program evaluation may not be as thorough or complete as a program evaluation incorporating a mixed methodology. The validity of qualitative methods may lead to more concrete, intimate, and profound conclusions and findings rather than purely numerical results which tend to be impersonal and restricted.

According to Rao and Woolcock (2003), significant issues relating to beliefs, perceptions, and identities "cannot be meaningfully reduced to numbers or adequately understood" in a purely numeric, quantitative form. Qualitative methods can develop richer and more meaningful forms of research when studying these types of concepts. Moreover, qualitative researchers believe that this method provides additional and specific attention to context.

Program evaluations that are conducted using quantitative methods are served better when measurable data is available. For example, if one has data such as grade point average or any type of statistical data related to one's program evaluation that one is interested in assessing, quantitative methods may be more appropriate to one's study than qualitative methods. The two types of statistical data that one can use in a program evaluation are (1) inferential, and (2) descriptive. According to Wilde and Sockey (1995) "Descriptive statistics are those used to describe the population -- numbers, percentages, and averages. Inferential statistics are used when the evaluator wants to make a generalized statement about the importance of differences or similarities among groups" (Quantitative Analyses section, ¶ 2).

In contrast, process issues that are interpreted via a qualitative method can help researchers understand a particular impact of a situation more so than measuring that situation in a quantitative manner. Studies such as program evaluations looking at the value of a teacher education program dealing with interventions that need deep inquiry into issues relating to process may be more effectively evaluated with qualitative methods. Although, many researchers believe that a mixed methodology can provide multiple, important levels to one's program evaluation. An example of this will be discussed later in this paper where a mixed methodology is used to design an online undergraduate teacher education program. The hypothetical program evaluation seeks to identify and measure if an online undergraduate teacher education program effectively trained teachers.

Qualitative methods used in program evaluation have various disadvantages which include the following: (1) groups can often be selected by a personal peculiarity of the researcher or recommended by a participant (i.e. sampling known as "snowball"); and (2) since qualitative analysis is interpreted by the researcher's judgment, other researchers may interpret the same data differently unless the researcher uses a triangulation method (Rao & Woolcock, 2003, p. 169). Quantitative methods in program evaluation objectively measure and interpret data. Comparative case-study research is an example of quantitative measures deduced from a large number of qualitative responses such as when the number of cases is diminutive but the units of analysis are quite large (Rao & Woolcock, 2003, p. 169).

Comparing & Contrasting Qualitative & Quantitative Data Collection Methods

According to McNamara (2007), the following table outlines various methods used in program evaluation data collection and highlights areas such as overall purpose of a program evaluation, advantages, and challenges. In addition, the table compares and contrasts differences between qualitative and quantitative data collection methods used in program evaluations.

Table 3

Comparing & Contrasting Qualitative & Quantitative Data Collection Methods

Method	Overall Purpose	Advantages	Challenges
Questionnaires, surveys, checklists (quantitative)	when need to quickly and/or easily get lots of information from people in a non threatening way	-can complete anonymously -inexpensive to administer -easy to compare and analyze -administer to many people -can get lots of data -many sample questionnaires already exist	-might not get careful feedback -wording can bias client's responses -are impersonal -in surveys, may need sampling expert -doesn't get full story
Interviews (qualitative)	when want to fully understand someone's impressions or experiences, or learn more about their answers to questionnaires	-get full range and depth of information -develops relationship with client -can be flexible with client	-can take much time -can be hard to analyze and compare -can be costly -interviewer can bias client's responses
Documentation review (quantitative)	when want impression of how program operates without interrupting the	-get comprehensive and historical information -doesn't interrupt	-often takes much time -info may be incomplete -need to be quite clear

	program; is from review of applications, finances, memos, minutes, etc.	program or client's routine in program -information already exists -few biases about information	about what looking for -not flexible means to get data; data restricted to what already exists
Observation (qualitative)	to gather accurate information about how a program actually operates, particularly about processes	-view operations of a program as they are actually occurring -can adapt to events as they occur	-can be difficult to interpret seen behaviors -can be complex to categorize observations -can influence behaviors of program participants -can be expensive
focus groups (qualitative)	explore a topic in depth through group discussion, e.g., about reactions to an experience or suggestion, understanding common complaints, etc.; useful in evaluation and marketing	-quickly and reliably get common impressions -can be efficient way to get much range and depth of information in short time -can convey key information	-can be hard to analyze responses -need good facilitator for safety and closure -difficult to schedule 6-8 people together

		about programs	
Case studies (qualitative)	to fully understand or depict client's experiences in a program, and conduct comprehensive examination through cross comparison of cases	-fully depicts client's experience in program input, process and results -powerful means to portray program to outsiders	-usually quite time consuming to collect, organize and describe -represents depth of information, rather than breadth

From "Basic Guide to Program Evaluation," by C. McNamara, 2007.

Regardless of which research methodology one chooses to use in a program evaluation, many program evaluations require a quick turnaround with clear and unambiguous policy recommendations. For these reason, a mixed methodology may be more time consuming and costly than if one were to use either one or the other research method only. Although, a mixed methodology used in program evaluation could provide more comprehensive findings. According to McNamara (2007), "the evaluator uses a combination of methods, for example, a questionnaire to quickly collect a great deal of information from a lot of people, and then interviews to get more in-depth information from certain respondents to the questionnaires" (Overall Goal in Selecting Methods section, ¶ 2). Many researchers believe using both quantitative and qualitative methods combined is the best way to reach reliability. In this way, triangulation can be achieved by comparing and contrasting the data complied and reported.

Data Collection

Qualitative researchers who are experienced and adept at data collection via interview process or group discussion may find more accurate results in his or her study than an inexperienced researcher or interviewer using a well-structured, quantitative survey. Regardless of which methodology a researcher chooses to use in his or her study, one's questions and problem should direct which methodology one decides to use. Furthermore, researchers need to be cognizant of the appearance of subjectivity and should seek to provide results that are as objective as possible so that one's study is viewed as relevant to one's research community. Finally, researchers must be aware of the limitations and advantages of each type of methodology employed in program evaluation to best accommodate one's study in meaningful and germane ways.

Reliability, Validity, & Ethics

> ## Conducting Research
> - The two most important issues when conducting research are reliability and validity.
> - Reliability occurs when the research produces the same results each time they are applied to the same issue.
> - Essentially, the research produces consistent results.

The evaluation methodology can include qualitative, narrative interviews conducted by the researcher and data collected from various reports, medical documents, Internet research, books, case studies, and peer-reviewed studies. Quantitative data can be compiled via statistics reported by the evaluated system, program, governing agencies, and various other reporting agencies not associated with the system or program operators. Reliability, validity, and ethical considerations are addressed in the following manner:

Example of Data Collection

Example of Data Collection from a Recent Study I Conducted that can be used as a Guide or Model for your Evaluation:

Data Collection

Many factors were involved in the consideration of appropriate research methods for data collection and instrumentation (Anderson & Kanuka, 2003; Church & Waclawski, 1998; De Vellis, 2003; Laub, 2003; Miles & Huberman, 1994; Page, 2005). The factors included the need for data from subject matter experts based upon lived experiences, access to a representative population, and varied perspectives from diverse participants.

Creswell (2002) identified observations, interviews, documents, and audiovisual materials as forms of data collection. Unstructured observational data in different venues as a participant observer or non-participant observer were not available, and this precluded the opportunity to take field notes or to record data to inform the research. The most appropriate and available data collection method to achieve data validity and reliability in the target population frame was the semistructured interview (Elliott, 2005).

This research study utilized telephone interviews to capture a wider range of participants in terms of geographic locations. The telephone interviews using semistructured questions provided the most appropriate instrument to understand the central phenomenon of online teaching because most of the emphasis was on the role of the researcher to elicit and represent an interpretive relationship of the world (Hiller & DiLuzio, 2004). Telephone interviews, however, permit less time to collect data but allow better access to research participants, especially for those in different geographic locations. Thus, this research study utilized telephone interviews. Participants were informed that the conversation would be recorded and would be transcribed for data analysis. The interviews lasted approximately 20 to 30 minutes, and interviews took place only once.

For the purpose of this study, the qualitative interview participants were initiated by the researcher and were also nominated by those that knew their online work and were responding as individuals, not faculty, at a specific institution. In fact, some did not have any institutional affiliation whatsoever. The researcher invited online faculty such as colleagues and acquaintances to participate based upon their years of experience in the field of online teaching in the college of education at various institutions. Instructions as to how to participate in the study were made available. Interested participants received an overview of the study. If their qualifications matched the criteria considered in this study, they were included as potential participants. All potential participants were contacted to arrange for telephone interviews. Consent forms were sent prior to the scheduled interview session. The informed consent form had to be returned prior to the actual interview process. During the interview process, participants were informed that audio tapes were to be employed to ensure that their responses could be transcribed appropriately. A transcribed copy was also provided to each participant for approval after the interview process. The data collection process ended when the researcher received the approved copy of the transcribed interview. After that, the data was inputted to the NVivo© qualitative analysis software program for data analysis.

Instrumentation

Qualitative research uses different tools, instruments, and methods to collect and assemble data; the primary tool necessary to carry out qualitative research, however, is the researcher (Marshall & Rossman, 1999). Interviews allow the researcher to describe and capture complex discursive activities that produce meaning to the respondent, with interviews being a traditional qualitative approach (Hiller & DiLuzio, 2004). The research strategy that was used was a semi-structured interview conducted with a purposive sample of the research participants from the represented sectors. All interviews used a series of guided questions, were conducted by telephone, and were electronically recorded on audio tape; the results were professionally transcribed to ensure accuracy. The semi-structured interview questions had been developed according to the research questions posed for this study. In addition the semi-structured interview questions had undergone field testing by three experts for filtering before being used for the final interviews. Each question was delivered in the same manner for all interviewees. Each participant was provided with a compact disc of the recorded interview and a copy of the transcription within two weeks of the date of the interview, in order for participants to have an opportunity to review, append, comment, or modify the original responses to the question prior to the information being used as a basis of data analysis.

The interviews were evaluated for content analysis using the NVivo© qualitative analysis software program to identify significant elements relating to importance and unobtrusive themes (Godau, 2004). Data that was gathered from the transcribed interviews was coded to reduce attributions to the component elements of cause, outcome, and links between cause and outcome. Coding was guided by the Leeds Attribution Coding Systems (Munton, Silvester, Stratton, & Hanks, 1999). The six stages of attributional coding included the following:

1. Source identification;
2. Extract attributions from transcripts;
3. Separate cause and outcome elements of the attributions;
4. Code speaker, agent or cause of the attribution, and target of the outcome;
5. Coding attributions on causal dimensions;
6. Analysis.

The causal dimensions included Stable or Unstable, Global or Specific, Internal or External, Personal or Universal, and Controllable or Uncontrollable. Attributional coding provided a means for providing sense-making in organizations but required time-consuming transcribed interviews for data. The objective was to identify manifest content for the elements that were physically present and countable from the interviews (Berg, 2001). The intent was to analyze the data and establish common themes, patterns, terms, or ideas that could inform a deeper understanding of the issue surrounding the research problem while articulating a rich description of the issue of online teaching (Elliott, 2005).

Data Analysis

The semi-structured interview questions for the research were based on the research questions to be addressed by the study. The interviews were conducted by telephone, recorded, and transcribed to ensure accuracy and verifiability. The interviews were evaluated for content analysis using NVivo©qualitative software to identify significant elements or manifested themes and explore any emergent attributes of online teaching experiences. The objective was to identify the manifest content for the elements that were physically present and countable from the interviews. The combined sources of research data were appropriate to the research design and strategy to obtain valid and reliable empirical information. Moustakas (1994) identified a modification of the van Kaam (1959) method of analysis. This was carried out for this study. The steps for analyzing the data from each participant's interview included the following (Moustakas, 1994):

1. Listing and preliminary grouping of every relevant experience.
2. Reduction and elimination of extraneous data to capture essential constituents of the phenomenon.
3. Clustering and identifying the invariant constituents to identify core themes of the experience.
4. Final identification and verification against the complete record of the research participant to ensure explicit relevancy and compatibility.
5. Construction for each co-researcher of an individualized textural description of the

experience based upon the verbatim transcripts using relevant and valid invariant constituents and themes.
6. Construction for each co-researcher of an individual structural description of the experience based upon individual textural description and imaginative variation.
7. Construction for each participant of a textural-structural description of the meaning and essence of the experiences. (pp. 120-122)

These steps were used for this qualitative study in order to ensure that the participants gathered would be able to express their lived experiences and that the data would be understood and interpreted accordingly. These steps allowed the development of a composite description of meaning and essence of experiences representing the population in order to draw generalizations which would help achieve the goals of the study.

Specifically, the following procedures were used to analyze the data:

Procedure #1: Listen to the interview tapes while reviewing interview transcriptions in order to validate accuracy of transcriptions. A reputable transcription service was used that commonly dealt with clients where confidentiality and anonymity were required (Thomae, 1999).

Procedure #2: Identify meaning units and assign appropriate idiographic themes. Idiographics involves the study of, explanation of, or interpretation of individual events or cases (Thomae, 1999).

Procedure #3: Compile similar idiographic themes into nomothetic themes. Nomothetic involves or pertains to the study or development of general or universal laws (Thomae, 1999).

Procedure #4: Group two or more similar nomothetic themes into clusters of related themes (Thomae, 1999).

Procedure #5: Report nomothetic themes in hierarchy order (Thomae, 1999).

Procedure #6: Create descriptive essays for the most popular themes and clusters (Thomae, 1999).

Procedure #7: Create a descriptive profile for all participants and their corresponding themes (Thomae, 1999).

The study was analyzed using triangulation techniques, which included the use of multiple data collection methods, analysts, data sources, or theories as collaborative evidence for the validity of standard qualitative research findings (Gall, Gall, & Borg, 2003, p. 640). For the study, multiple methods employed included qualitative analysis as well as the use of multiple analysts in the development of the qualitative component.

The triangulation method condensed, clustered, and sorted the data by implementing the following steps:

Step #1: Interview participants were selected in the following order: (a) three participants from a public university, (b) three participants from a private university, (c) three participants from a for-profit university, and (d) three participants from a research 1 university to triangulate how participants from four different types of institutions respond to the qualitative questions.

Step #2: Interview participants via phone with qualitative questions.

Step #3: Transcribe and give responses to the participants for review and approval.

Step #4: Collaborate with outside evaluator on the study to evaluate the transcriptions. Outside evaluator will collaborate to identify and analyze meaning units and assign themes (Creswell, 1998).

Validity

Creswell (2002) defined validity as the ability of the researcher to "draw meaningful and justifiable inferences from scores about the sample or population" (p. 651). Hammersley (1990) stated that validity was "the extent to which an account accurately represents the social phenomenon to which it refers" (p. 57). Validity is categorized into internal and external validity. Each type of validity has potential threats that can undermine the use of the research data (Golafshani, 2003).

Internal Validity

The passage of time between the beginning of the research and the conclusion without demonstrable progress, participating individuals changing during the process of the data collection, or a biased selection of the research population can all threaten internal validity. Measures were incorporated in the research to protect against potential internal threats to validity by gathering recommendations from experts in choosing participants that had lived experiences regarding online teaching. This established credibility and avoided potential biases. A number of features were used to encourage participants to remain engaged throughout the research process, including timely, personal, and courteous telephone contact, e-mails, and letters by the researcher. To avoid the researcher's possible bias as she fit the criteria necessary for those chosen for the study, she approached the telephone interviews by setting aside personal biases and ideas about online programs and online faculty's experiences and perceptions. In addition, she set aside possible bias as she collected and analyzed data. The researcher did not coach the participants, did not lead them in one direction or another, did not offer suggestions or comments regarding the responses, and only asked the interview questions without interjecting her opinions, beliefs, or viewpoints. As the data were collected and analyzed, the researcher collaborated with an outside evaluator.

The researcher mitigated any potential conflict of interest by not personally or professionally knowing any of the participants chosen for this study. There was no conflict of interest. The researcher is only employed as an online instructor and does not associate with other faculty members whatsoever as her working and teaching environment is isolated from other faculty members. She does not associate, have conversations, develop relationships, or work closely with other online faculty members. There was little to no personal bias or conflict of interest as the researcher has not worked with any of the faculty or had any discussions with them previous to the qualitative interviews conducted.

The research was conducted in a timely fashion in order to obviate any threats of data becoming irrelevant. The collection of data, through the recording of semistructured interviews, was anonymous and confidential, preventing the potential for any undue influence by any one research participant. The confidential and anonymous collection of data assisted in establishing trust with each research participant while enhancing the dependability of the data. Informed consent, confidentiality, and the protection of all recorded interviews using a unique numeric code to identify participants were measured. This provided the means to maintain internal validity and establish credibility based upon integrity (Hoepfl, 1997). All participants were provided the opportunity to terminate the interview at any point and to confirm the accuracy of each interview, which was transcribed after being recorded. Confirmation by the participants ensured that statements provided tacit assumptions of authenticity, objectivity, and accuracy to substantiate validity and reliability (Roberts & Priest, 2006).

External Validity

Neuman (2003) defined external validity as "the ability to generalize experimental findings to events and settings outside the experiment itself" (p. 255). Issues that affect the ability to draw correct inference from the sample data to other persons and settings can threaten external validity. Threats to external validity relate to applying the research findings to other contexts and situations. The use of subject matter experts can assist in promoting external validity. Expertise and agreement can frame the essential elements of tacit knowledge and mitigate challenges to external validity. Collection of data from participants in various and distinct faculty domains assisted in establishing external validity of the research findings for this study (Denzin & Lincoln, 2005, 2012).

Informed Consent

Gaining the trust and support of research participants is critical to informed and ethical academic inquiry and phenomenological researches (Marshall & Rossman, 1999; Walker, 2007). All participants were given an informed consent cover letter before scheduling interviews and participating in the research process. Participants were given the option to sign the consent forms manually or electronically. Participants provided their names for the consent forms. Consent forms including such personal information as the participant's name, phone number, and e-mail address were to be kept confidential by remaining in a locked, undisclosed location for a minimum of three years. After the minimum time, the consent forms and other documents associated with the participants were to be discarded through shredding. The purpose of the informed consent letter was to introduce the research effort, provide contact information, articulate the intent of the study, request voluntary participation by the recipients, and identify the anticipated information that participants would be expected to provide. Personal assurances of a committed participation, prompt scheduling of the interviews, and personal contact would diminish attrition and non-responsiveness and would ensure participation adequate to achieve thematic saturation.

Confidentiality

The informed consent letter articulated the procedural steps to maintain privacy, confidentiality, and the non-attribution of individual responses. The informed consent letter declared that the participant's background information would remain confidential and would not be released without prior expressed personal approval. Restricted access based upon a need to know would protect and secure participant information to maintain confidentiality and anonymity and ensure that all responses were secure from inappropriate disclosure, to enhance reliability and validity of provided data. All participants were required to sign and return the letter of consent to the researcher before participating in the research. All responses were secured in a locked repository and were to be maintained for three years after the conclusion of the research. All research data were to be destroyed after three years, with destruction conducted by shredding.

Participants were informed of the audio tapes that would be used in the interviews as a means to gather more detailed information. Participants were told that privacy and confidentiality of the participant in the research study would be respected. Confidentiality refers to the treatment of information that a participant disclosed in a relationship of trust, with the expectation that the information would not be divulged to others without permission from the participant (Johnson & Christensen, 2008).

DATA ANALYSIS & INTERPRETATION

Example of Quantitative Program Evaluation Data
An example of quantitative program evaluation data could be items such as grade point average or student evaluations. Underlying assumptions associated with quantitative methods include the following: (1) reality is objective, independent from the researcher, can be studied objectively; (2) researcher is separate and removed from those being researched; (3) research is value-free, values of the researcher are not part of the research; (4) research is constructed on deduction, logic, theories, and hypotheses, research is tested in a cause and effect manner; and (5) quantitative methods seek to develop generalizations contributing to theory enabling the researcher to understand a particular phenomenon, and explain, or predict (Dobbin & Gatowski, 1999).

According to Powell (2006), typical quantitative program evaluation methods include the following: (1) correlation, (2) concept mapping, (3) time series analysis, (4) meta-analysis, (5) cross-sectional design, (6) regression analysis, (7) matrix sampling, (8) panel studies, and (9) standardized tests. Quantitative methods in program evaluation are useful when researchers need to analyze and interpret statistical data and if this data is available and happens to meet the objective of the study. Education programs that need to address if standards are being met, could employ this methodology if narrative, opinions, views, and perceptions are not relevant to the study. Later in this paper, an example of how one might use quantitative methods in program evaluation will be discussed. The quantitative method takes the form of an online survey that is a forced choice, four-point, Likert-like scale with the following choices: excellent, good, fair, and poor.

Qualitative Research Approaches to Program Evaluation
Philosophy, Assumptions, & Components

> ## Data Analysis After Collection
> ## Summarizing
> - "the first time you sit down with your data is the only time you come to that particular set fresh"- Kratowohl.
>   - Reading and memoing
>   - Read write memos about field notes.
>   - Describing
>   - Develop comprehensive descriptions of setting, participants, etc.
>   - Classifying
>   - Breaking data into analytic units.
>   - Categories
>   - Themes

According to Onwuegbuzie and Leech (2007), qualitative researchers are interested in capturing "lived experiences" by means of text (p. 238). Furthermore, "in qualitative studies involving multiple cases, qualitative researchers must strike a fine balance between obtaining thick description from each case and obtaining comparative description from each comparison" (p. 249). Qualitative research involves a process of expressing words in a creative, expressive manner so that the complex views of those individuals studied are captured accurately (Creswell, p. 24, 1998). Qualitative research develops *how* or *what* types of questions then reduces the data one collects into themes or categories. From these themes and categories a narrative is developed. This narrative can take one of four forms which included a theory, a detailed view, or an abstract model (Creswell, p. 24, 1998).

From a global approach to qualitative methods, five traditions have been identified which include phenomenological studies, biography, case studies, grounded theory, and ethnographic studies. Qualitative research is most beneficial when one seeks knowledge that is complex, holistic, in-depth, and from the view of those being studied. These processes are described as fluid, illuminating, iterative, inductive, cumulative regarding developing findings and conclusions, validating, reinterpreting challenging data for reduction, and verification (Young, 2007, p. 5).

Participatory methods in program evaluation involve group participation from those individuals being studied. Participatory methodology for program evaluation includes three specific forms which include the interview technique, focus-groups, and key-informant interview. The researcher oftentimes can be directly involved in this form of qualitative methodology and may steer discussion in meaningful directions. Participatory methodology can convey significant and realistic impressions of individuals' experiences, lives, and situations in a way that allows outsiders a more accurate picture of the reality that these individuals are experiencing. Numerical data may not represent these types of studies in the best possible manner whereas a participatory, qualitative methodology is better suited.

Focus- groups are another form of qualitative methodology that researchers can use that similarly involve a moderator directing smaller groups of individuals into consensus regarding a particular issue being addressed in the study. Each of these methods employs the interview technique to collect data. According Rao and Woolcock (2003), "Another important qualitative technique that uses interview methods is the key-informant interview, which is an extended one-on-one exchange with someone who is a leader or unique in some way that is relevant to the study" (p. 171). In each of these cases, the researcher can be involved in more direct ways as a participant of the study or in less direct manners such as a short-termed, detached, distant, observer. Participatory methods can be used effectively in higher education program evaluation when for example; faculty, administrators, or staff need to be involved in meaningful ways that address change or transformation. In addition, this methodology can be useful if narrative views, opinions, and perceptions are relevant to the study.

According to Rao and Woolcock (2003), when a qualitative approach is used alone, faulty and subjective conclusions could be a result. A combination of quantitative and qualitative methods could provide a more integrated study with more accurate, precise, and objective findings. The appearance of subjectivity in one's study can be a challenge when one uses mainly qualitative methods such as these in program evaluation. Although, using only a qualitative approach in program evaluation may prove to be necessary depending upon the nature of one's study and the type of problem statement being addressed.

Qualitative methods can identify "unobservables" which can be made observable through field investigations and focus-group discussions (Rao & Woolcock, 2003, p. 186). At times, one's study must incorporate only qualitative methods as this may be the best manner in which to address one's questions and problem. The following table lists various underlying assumptions associated with qualitative methods.

Quantitative/Qualitative Data

- Qualitative data: non-numerical measures
    - Verbal feedback, narratives, open-ended feedback
    - Analyzed from a context viewpoint
    - Usually informs process evaluation
- Mixed methods evaluations utilize quantitative and qualitative data

Table 4
Underlying Assumptions of Qualitative Methods

many realities can exist in all circumstances, i.e. the researcher, participants being studied, and the audience or reader of the study; many representations are included in the research;
researcher interacts with participants of the study, researcher assertively involves himself or herself in the study, researcher tries to reduce distance between himself or herself and the individuals being studied;
the researcher clearly recognizes and validates the worth of the research; research is context-bound;
inductive forms of logic define the research; components of the research originate from the respondents or those being studied rather than being established by the researcher; the purpose of the study is to reveal and disclose theories or patterns that assist in clarifying phenomenon;
triangulating - a gathering of information comes from various and multiple sources.

From "A Judge's Deskbook on the Basic Philosophies and Methods of Science: Model Curriculum," by S. A. Dobbin and S. I. Gatowski, 1999.

Indicators & Standards

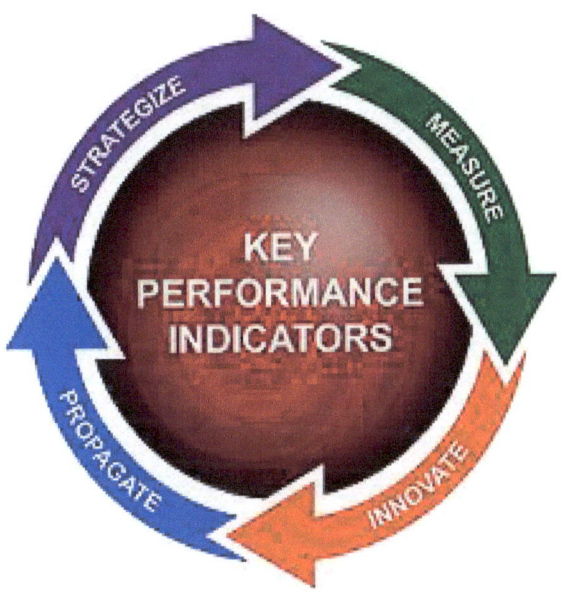

What are some measurable or observable elements that can tell you about the performance of the program being evaluated?

Various types of measurable or observable elements in a program evaluation can include: (1) portfolios, (2) role-play, (3) critiques, (4) formative, (5) summative, (6) journal, (7) formal papers, (8) essays, (9) concept mapping, (10) oral questioning, (11) audio taping, (12) video taping, (13) group work, and (14) peer learning (Bahous & Nabhani, 2011; Brown & McIlroy, 2011; Decelle & Sherrod, 2011; Dickerson, 2011; Portugal, 2015).

A program evaluation can include many of these elements when available and appropriate to the needs of the evaluation. In addition, a variety of these assessment tools might be used based upon the ability level and learning styles of the participants. Various measures can be used to address a differentiated approach to measurement and assessment while accommodating participants and outside evaluators (Bahous & Nabhani, 2011; Brown & McIlroy, 2011; Decelle & Sherrod, 2011; Dickerson, 2011; Portugal, 2015).

What constitutes "success"? (i.e. by what standards will you compare your evaluation findings?)

One can use various outside evaluators with specific expertise and experiences in the topic areas and content assessed and measured in a program evaluation. Triangulation measures can be used based on these outside evaluators' expertise. The additions of their experiences and expertise to the project can be triangulated to form conclusions, suggestions, findings, and improvement measures. A program evaluation does not need to be performed in a vacuum, but rather can incorporate the expertise of outside evaluators throughout the process.

Data Collection & Analysis

> **Conducting Program Evaluation: Gather Data**
>
> 4. Gather the data.
>   - What information do you need in order to answer your question?
>   - Use multiple sources of data, or multiple outcome measures, wherever possible (triangulation).
>   - Decide whether you need to consider student achievement data, psychosocial data, career data, school data, process data, perception data, and/or results data.

For data collection, the lived experiences and expertise of participants and evaluators can be documented in the various manners listed above. Interviews, observations, documents, audio and visual materials can be collected for an evaluation. Non-participant observer and participant observer unstructured observational data from various venues can be collected as well. Telephone interviews can be transcribed and NVivo qualitative analysis instrumentation can be used to identify common themes and coded for findings interpretation. (Portugal, 2015).

USE, COMMUNICATION, & EVALUATION

The assessment and evaluation of clinical performance should also be inspected. The process of the actual evaluation is another factor. Fair and reasonable evaluation can be a challenge and ethical consideration as well as form and process considerations are necessary. The use of appropriate communication tools should be considered when meeting with stakeholders and disseminating.

Use

What actions will be taken to promote evaluation use?

To promote evaluation use and implementation of suggestions for improvement, the following ideas could assist:

1. Workshops,
2. Training,
3. Curriculum creation,
4. Curriculum revisions,
5. Online modules, tutorials,
6. The use of outside experts,
7. The use of outside monitors,
8. Revised standards, objectives, goals, or
9. Development of new processes, procedures, standards, objectives, goals
10. Clinical conferences,
11. Case discussions, and
12. The creation of self-evaluation, self-reflection, and ethical measuring tools (Portugal, 2017).

How will evaluation findings be used?

Evaluation findings should be used to inform, educate, alert the public, improve positive changes, improve services, improve patient care, improve educational services to stakeholders, and improve communication processes.

Who is responsible for implementing evaluation recommendations?

Relevant experts and participants can help develop suggestions for improvement and help disseminate the recommendations within their communities and sphere of influence. Recommendations can be made by both formative and summative evaluations. Typically, the burden of a summative report might have two challenges to overcome: (1) general acceptance, and (2) await implementation until a future program (The Electoral Knowledge Network: ACE, 2017). The creation and communication of findings, suggestions, and recommendations is essential to evaluation success. Recommendations that are not viewed as important, serious, and valued can affect forthcoming work. With these challenges, a program evaluation could be in vain. "Surprisingly, a report that merely describes the impact of the programme is not always well-received" (The Electoral Knowledge Network: ACE, 2017). Recognition, affirmation, "buy-in," and suggestions for improvements are components necessary for program evaluation success.

Communication

Which evaluation stakeholders will you communicate with and why (e.g., update on status of evaluation, invite to meetings, share interim or final findings)?

Relevant participants and experts as well as those within their sphere of influence can be part of the updates on the status of evaluation.

What methods (e.g., in-person meetings, emails, written reports, presentations) will you use to communicate with evaluation stakeholders?

The following presentation methods can be developed:

1. Power Point presentations,
2. Prezi presentations,
3. Audio - visual presentations,
4. professional development workshops,
5. Conferences (one-on-one and / or groups),
6. Curriculum development,
7. Written manuals, reports, charts, data facts sheets can be distributed to various stakeholders depending on their specific needs,
8. Email,
9. ListServs,
10. Newsletters: community, internal and / or external,
11. Publication: public, official, governmental, state, federal, corporate, internal and / or external, books, peer-reviewed articles, internal and / or external websites.

Why are these methods appropriate for the specific evaluation stakeholder audience of interest?

Various methods should be used to communicate and share findings and suggestions for improvement to reach a variety of groups and stakeholders with different needs. In addition, consideration for differentiated instructional models should be applied such as ability levels, learning styles, multi-generational factors, cultural factors, diversity, technology integration, Andragogy Theory, best practices, Cognitive Dissonance Theory, intrinsic and extrinsic motivational factors, student agency, personalized learning, personalized feedback, student-centered learning theory, engagement techniques, and Behaviorist, Cognitive, Socio-Cultural Theories (Portugal, 2017; Portugal, 2015a; Portugal, 2015b; Portugal, 2015c; Portugal, 2015d; Portugal, 2014e).

Evaluating the Evaluation

How will you evaluate the evaluation? (Instruments? Stakeholder input? Data analysis?)

A final conference can be held for stakeholders where communication can take place about the evaluation process, findings, data analysis reported. In addition, the program site can be evaluated based on how well the needs of stakeholders and services provided met expectations, goals, and objectives. Was the philosophy of the evaluated congruent with stakeholder needs? Was the opportunity to meet all objectives given? A preparation phase for the evaluation should involve a continuous quality improvement process. Important considerations include attention to structure, process, and outcomes. Stakeholders should be provided a means for critical reflection of their future roles when a clinical performance evaluation has taken place.

Template Using Quantitative & Qualitative Approaches to Program Evaluation

A program evaluation is a technical report that consists of various and specific components. According to the literature, a program evaluation contains the following components that are sequenced in order and described:

1. Title page.
2. Executive summary -one or two pages including subheadings listed below:
    a. Introduction and background - introduce the evaluation and provide background information about the program one is evaluating.
    b. Guiding questions - describe the focus of the evaluation (needs, process, or output), then state the questions one identifies that one wants to answer in bullet statements.
    c. Evaluation methods- describe the methods one used to collect and analyze the data to answer the questions one identified.
    d. Key findings - an introductory brief paragraph in bullets that leads the reader and lists key findings.

e. Conclusion - summarize the evaluation's conclusion.
   f. Key recommendations - an introductory paragraph leading the reader and listing key recommendations in bullets.
3. Introduction and background - introduce reader to the evaluation and incorporate the following subheadings:
   a. Purpose of the program or project - provide background information about the program that one is evaluating to familiarize the reader with the program.
   b. Purpose and aim of the evaluation - describe why the evaluation was conducted, who one's audience was, what they generally wanted to know, and why.
   c. Guiding evaluation questions:
      i. Describe which of the three types of evaluation was conducted (needs assessment based, process-based, or outcomes-based).
      ii. Write a stem sentence that leads the reader to the guiding questions.
      iii. List the evaluation questions one wishes to answer in the evaluation.
   d. Goals and objectives of the evaluation - describe the goal of the evaluation and the activities one conducted to complete it.
   e. Evaluator relationship to the program - describe one's relationship to the program and how one came to be connected to the program. Is one an internal member or an external member. Describe one's work with

stakeholders to develop the focus of the evaluation and the questions themselves.
  f. Rationale for selection of the program – describe the "why" of the program and the focus of the evaluation selected for examination; what was there about the program that made one's choice important.
4. Evaluation methodology:
   a. Research design:
      i. Describe the type of the evaluation: summative or formative and why.
      ii. Describe the nature of the evaluation: needs assessment, process monitoring, or outcome. Describe what the choice is and why that choice was made.
      iii. Describe the evaluation approach: management-oriented, program improvement-oriented, objectives-oriented, and why.
      iv. Describe the type of methodology(ies) that one is going to use to answer one's guiding questions. Identify and describe the methodology(ies) used in the evaluation (i.e. mixed, qualitative, quantitative). If one used a quantitative method, did one use a close-ended survey. If one used a qualitative method, did one conduct interviews with open-ended questions or field observation. If one used mixed methods, which methods did one mix and did one use a component design (triangulation, complementary

and expansion) or an integrated design (iterative-spiral, embedded, holistic, transformative) to "mix" the data. Present a rationale for selecting this particular methodology(ies). Address each such as describing one's instrumentation; did one use a questionnaire, interview, focus group, pre-existing records, test scores, other ratings and measurements, or multiple methods e.g. combination of questionnaire and interviews. Attach the actual instruments, interview questions, and focus group protocols in the paper's appendix.
b. Sample and setting - describe who was included and excluded in the evaluation and how were they chosen. What kind of sampling method was used: random sample, purposive sample, cluster sample, or stratified sample. Who are they. What is their number. What are their jobs or functions. What titles do they hold. What type of setting are they in. What environment is one operating in to conduct the evaluation process.
c. Data collection - describe how one collected the data to answer one's guiding questions.
d. Measurement methods - describe the measurement methods that one used in the data collection process. If one is collecting data with a questionnaire, what type of rating scale is one using. For example, a

Likert scale from one through five that measures "strongly agree" to "strongly disagree" can be used. If one is using qualitative methods, how will one measure what one is collecting.

e. Data analysis - describe how one is going to analyze or interpret the data, once collected, to make it meaningful to one's audience to answer one's guiding questions. For example, if one is going to use a questionnaire that results in gathering numbers of responses (quantitative) on a Likert scale, will one compile all the answers and conduct a "frequency tabulation" analysis using SPSS to see how often a certain response to a question occurred. If one is doing open-ended question interviews (qualitative), will one be doing a content analysis of the respondents' comments to determine trends. Once data is interpreted, the data is presented to one's audience through bar graphs, charts, and pie charts.

f. Protection of human rights - anytime one conducts an evaluation or research, one must think how one is going to protect the rights and privileges of those that one is interacting with and observing. This section describes how one will ensure this occurs.

g. Limits of design - no design or circumstance is perfect and limitations can influence the evaluation process. This section describes what the limits of the design were to inform

the reader. Was one not able to field test a questionnaire. Were the individuals unwilling to cooperate with one candidly. Did one have limited time to conduct interviews. This section will briefly state the things that are most important and that impacted one's evaluation.
   h. Best practices – this section will defend from the literature what the experts note, why one's choices were good ones, and why one chose his or her particular research design. This section will support the choices that one made in the design of the evaluation.
5. Findings - the findings are the heart of the evaluation report and use the interpreted data to answer each of one's guiding questions. Present the hard data first (data collected) under each question. If anything emerged from that question that one felt was thought provoking, enter that at the end of one's description of the findings for that question. This is called soft data.
   a. Question one: state the question:
      - Report the findings that relate to that question. This is where one answers the question and places whatever graphs and tables one has that relates to that particular question.
      - Did anything unanticipated emerge from one's efforts.
   b. Question two: state the question: follow same format as mentioned in question one.

      c. Question three: state the question: follow same format as mentioned in question one.
6. Summary discussion – this section will interpret the strengths and weaknesses of the program and interpret the results of the evaluation.
7. Recommendations - this section will make recommendations for program improvement and will discuss relevant next steps to take based upon the evaluation results.
8. References.
9. Appendices – attach survey questionnaire(s), interview questions, and additional instrumentation (Creswell, 1998; Fitzpatrick, Sanders, & Worthen, 2004; Gall, Gall, & Borg, 2003; McNamara, 2007; Sanders, 1994; Survedi & Morford, 2003; Wilde & Sockey, 1995).

Logic Model Charts

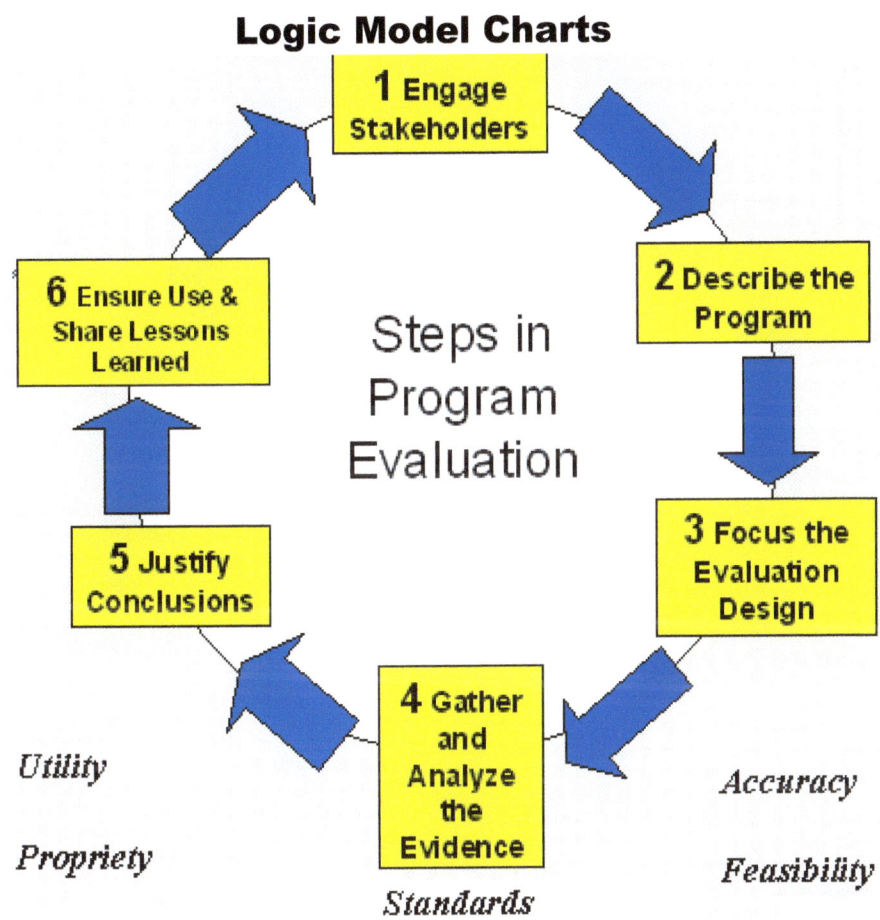

Steps of planning health education and intervention

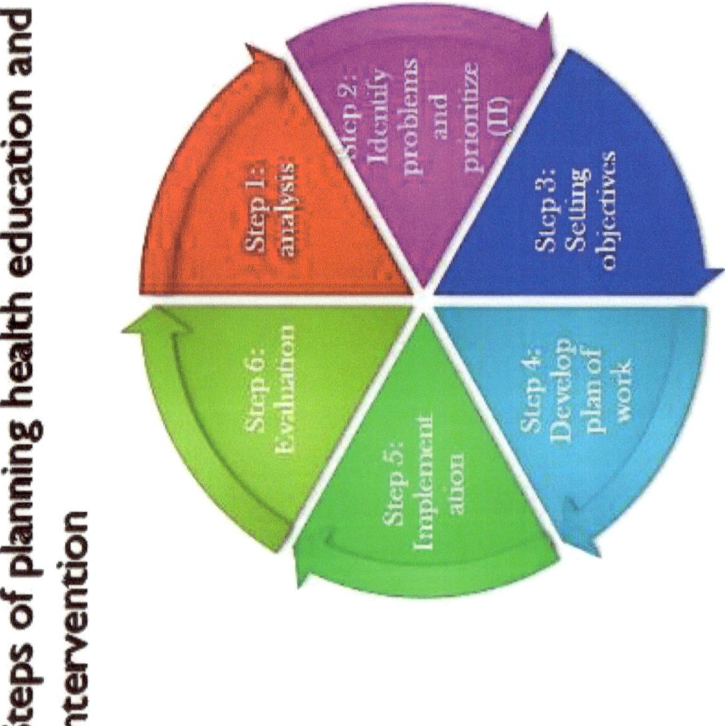

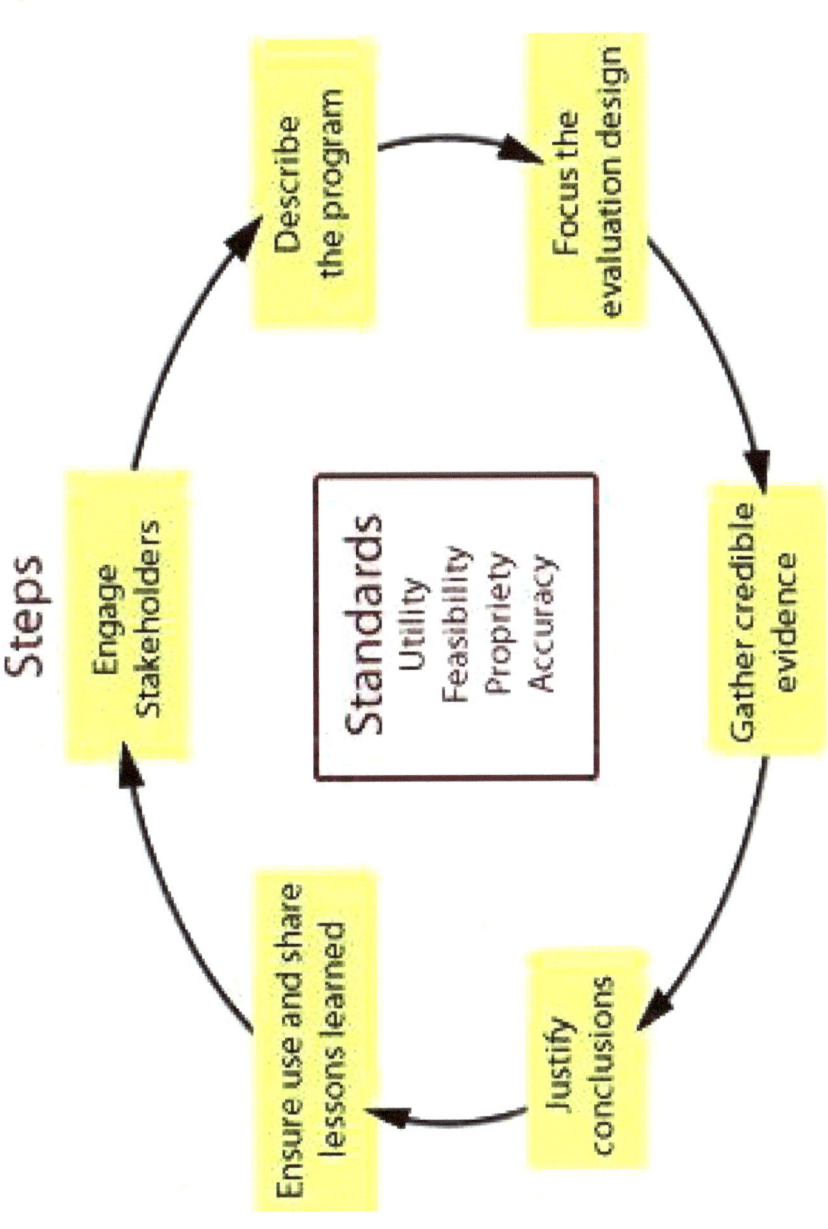

The six building blocks of a health system

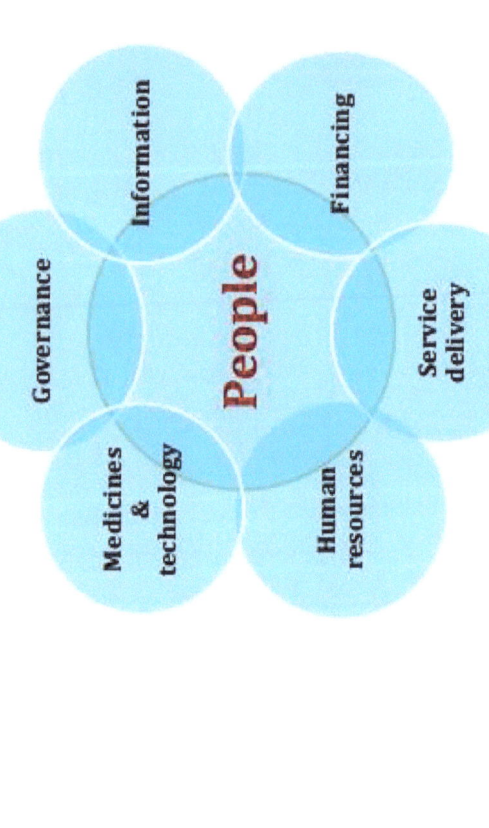

Elements of health systems interact together to form a complex system, and the health system interacts with the wider context within which it is situated. These interactions affect the achievement of goals for health systems.

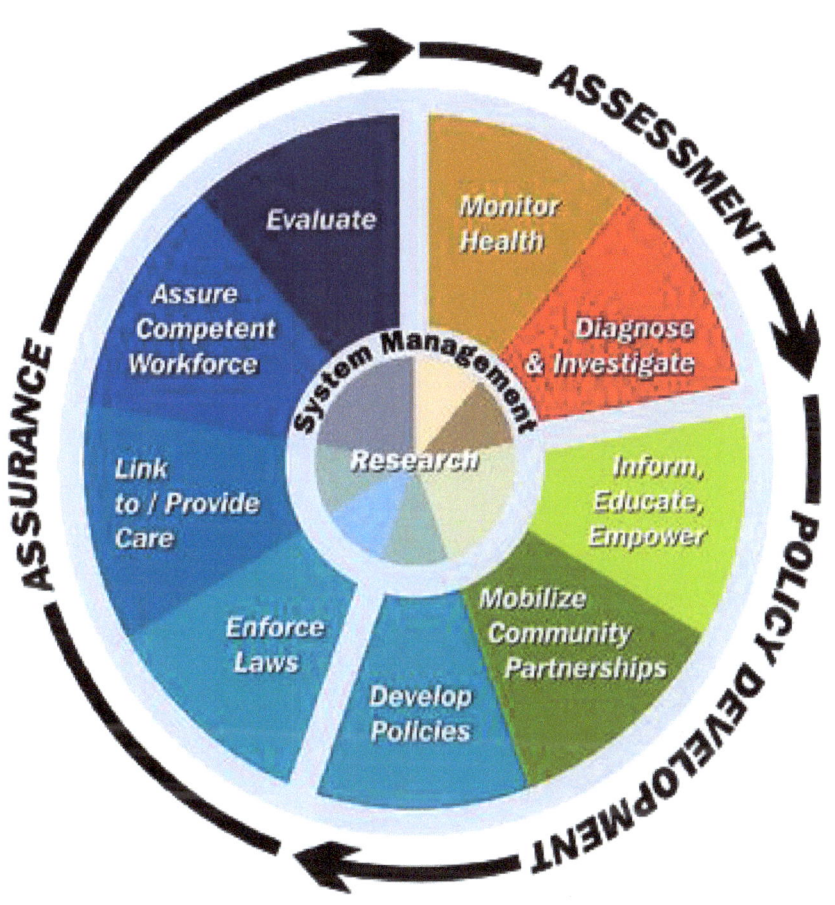

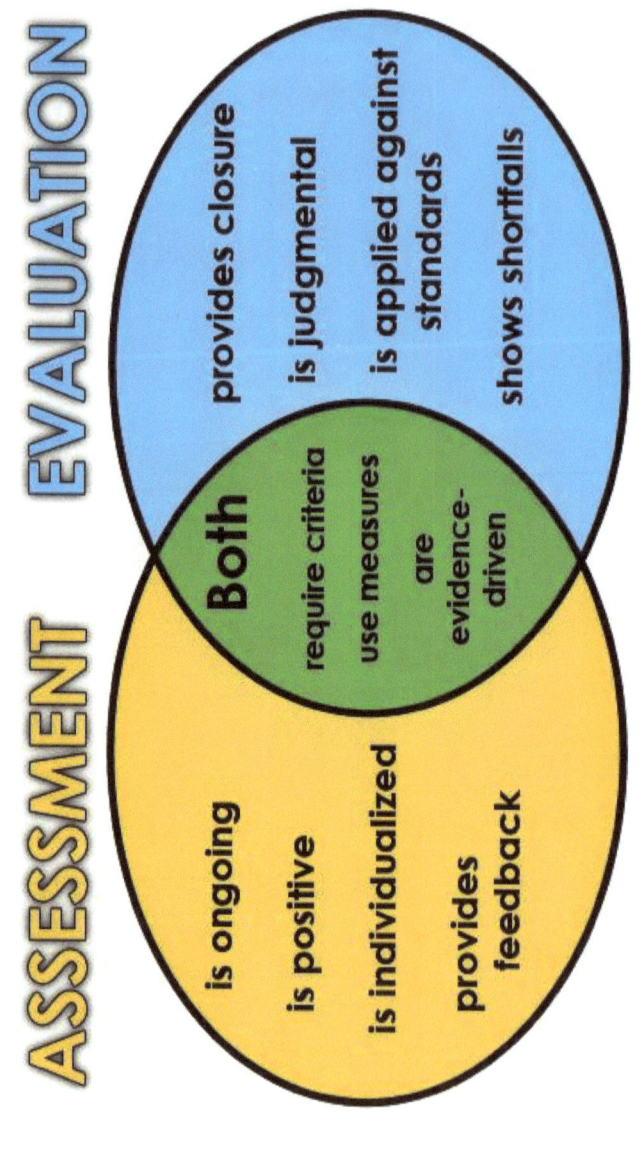

American College of Healthcare Executives (ACHE) Code of Ethics

PREAMBLE

The purpose of the Code of Ethics of the American College of Healthcare Executives is to serve as a standard of conduct for members. It contains standards of ethical behavior for healthcare executives in their professional relationships. These relationships include colleagues, patients or others served; members of the healthcare executive's organization and other organizations; the community; and society as a whole.

The Code of Ethics also incorporates standards of ethical behavior governing individual behavior, particularly when that conduct directly relates to the role and identity of the healthcare executive.

The fundamental objectives of the healthcare management profession are to maintain or enhance the overall quality of life, dignity and well-being of every individual needing healthcare service and to create an equitable, accessible, effective and efficient healthcare system.

Healthcare executives have an obligation to act in ways that will merit the trust, confidence and respect of healthcare professionals and the general public. Therefore, healthcare executives should lead lives that embody an exemplary system of values and ethics.

In fulfilling their commitments and obligations to patients or others served, healthcare executives function as moral advocates and models. Since every management decision affects the health and well-being of both individuals and communities, healthcare executives must carefully evaluate the possible outcomes of their decisions. In organizations that deliver healthcare services, they must work to safeguard and foster the rights, interests and prerogatives of patients or others served.

The role of moral advocate requires that healthcare executives take actions necessary to promote such rights, interests and prerogatives.
Being a model means that decisions and actions will reflect personal integrity and ethical leadership that others will seek to emulate.

I. THE HEALTHCARE EXECUTIVE'S RESPONSIBILITIES TO THE PROFESSION OF HEALTHCARE MANAGEMENT

The healthcare executive shall:

- Uphold the Code of Ethics and mission of the American College of Healthcare Executives;
- Conduct professional activities with honesty, integrity, respect, fairness and good faith in a manner that will reflect well upon the profession;
- Comply with all laws and regulations pertaining to healthcare management in the jurisdictions in which the healthcare executive is located or conducts professional activities;
- Maintain competence and proficiency in healthcare management by implementing a personal program

of assessment and continuing professional education;
- Avoid the improper exploitation of professional relationships for personal gain;
- Disclose when appropriate, avoid financial and other conflicts of interest;
- Use this Code to further the interests of the profession and not for selfish reasons;
- Respect professional confidences;
- Enhance the dignity and image of the healthcare management profession through positive public information programs; and
- Refrain from participating in any activity that demeans the credibility and dignity of the healthcare management profession.

II. THE HEALTHCARE EXECUTIVE'S RESPONSIBILITIES TO PATIENTS OR OTHERS SERVED

The healthcare executive shall, within the scope of his or her authority:

- Work to ensure the existence of a process to evaluate the quality of care or service rendered;
- Avoid practicing or facilitating discrimination and institute safeguards to prevent discriminatory organizational practices;
- Work to ensure the existence of a process that will advise patients or others served of the rights, opportunities, responsibilities and risks regarding available healthcare services;

- Work to ensure that there is a process in place to facilitate the resolution of conflicts that may arise when values of patients and their families differ from those of employees and physicians;
- Demonstrate zero tolerance for any abuse of power that compromises patients or others served;
- Work to provide a process that ensures the autonomy and self-determination of patients or others served;
- Work to ensure the existence of procedures that will safeguard the confidentiality and privacy of patients or others served; and
- H. Work to ensure the existence of an ongoing process and procedures to review, develop and consistently implement evidence-based clinical practices throughout the organization.

III. THE HEALTHCARE EXECUTIVE'S RESPONSIBILITIES TO THE ORGANIZATION

The healthcare executive shall, within the scope of his or her authority:

- Provide healthcare services consistent with available resources, and when there are limited resources, work to ensure the existence of a resource allocation process that considers ethical ramifications;
- Conduct both competitive and cooperative activities in ways that improve community healthcare services;

- Lead the organization in the use and improvement of standards of management and sound business practices;
- Respect the customs, beliefs and practices of patients or others served, consistent with the organization's philosophy;
- Be truthful in all forms of professional and organizational communication, and avoid disseminating information that is false, misleading or deceptive;
- Report negative financial and other information promptly and accurately, and initiate appropriate action;
- Prevent fraud and abuse and aggressive accounting practices that may result in disputable financial reports;
- Create an organizational environment in which both clinical and management mistakes are minimized and, when they do occur, are disclosed and addressed effectively;
- Implement an organizational code of ethics and monitor compliance; and
- Provide ethics resources and mechanisms for staff to address ethical organizational and clinical issues.

IV. THE HEALTHCARE EXECUTIVE'S RESPONSIBILITIES TO EMPLOYEES

Healthcare executives have ethical and professional obligations to the employees they manage that encompass but are not limited to:

- Creating a work environment that promotes ethical conduct;
- Providing a work environment that encourages a free expression of ethical concerns and provides mechanisms for discussing and addressing such concerns;
- Promoting a healthy work environment, which includes freedom from harassment, sexual and other, and coercion of any kind, especially to perform illegal or unethical acts;
- Promoting a culture of inclusivity that seeks to prevent discrimination on the basis of race, ethnicity, religion, gender, sexual orientation, age or disability;
- Providing a work environment that promotes the proper use of employees' knowledge and skills; and
- Providing a safe and healthy work environment.

V. THE HEALTHCARE EXECUTIVE'S RESPONSIBILITIES TO COMMUNITY AND SOCIETY

The healthcare executive shall:

- Work to identify and meet the healthcare needs of the community;
- Work to support access to healthcare services for all people;
- Encourage and participate in public dialogue on healthcare policy issues, and advocate solutions that will improve health status and promote quality healthcare;
- Apply short- and long-term assessments to management decisions affecting both community and society; and
- Provide prospective patients and others with adequate and accurate information, enabling them to make enlightened decisions regarding services.

VI. THE HEALTHCARE EXECUTIVE'S RESPONSIBILITY TO REPORT VIOLATIONS OF THE CODE

A member of ACHE who has reasonable grounds to believe that another member has violated this Code has a duty to communicate such facts to the Ethics Committee.

Conclusion

In closing, this book provides an example of how one might design a program evaluation of a health care system or education program. In addition, how to outline an evaluation and what components are involved based upon standard program evaluation methods were presented. Qualitative and quantitative research in program evaluation is described. Finally, underlying philosophy, assumptions, and components of quantitative and qualitative approaches to program evaluation was compared and contrasted with an appendix template provided.

Appendix
Program Evaluation Template

DESCRIPTION OF PROGRAM TO BE EVALUATED

This section provides detailed information about the health and wellness education program to be evaluated. This section describes the program, its history, the identified need the program is filling, context, and stakeholder engagement, including the target population.

Program Description and History

- What is the history of the selected health and wellness education program?
- What is the identified need for the program you are evaluating?
- What are the overall goals and outcomes of the program?
- How are the goals and outcomes currently measured?
- What are the program's major educational activities?
- What context/environment exists for the program to be evaluated?

Stakeholder Engagement
- Who are the stakeholders for this evaluation? (Identify at least three sets of stakeholders: (1) Individuals in charge of program operations, (2) target population served by the program including

demographics and need addressed by program, and individuals who will use the evaluation findings.)
- What role will they play in developing this evaluation plan?
- How do you plan to engage these stakeholders when implementing the evaluation plan (e.g., participate in collecting data, help to interpret findings)?

Note: You may either complete the table or write a paragraph for this item.

Stakeholder Engagement Plan (Add cells as needed)

Stakeholder Group	Interest or Perspective	Role in the Evaluation	How and When to Engage

PURPOSE & LOGIC MODEL

For this section of the evaluation proposal, you will identify the evaluation purpose and develop a logic model (graphical depiction) of the program you plan to evaluate. The logic model will provide information on inputs, activities, outputs, and outcomes. <u>A logic model template is provided through a link on the assignment page.</u> You will also address the proposed timeline and potential evaluation budget.

Evaluation Purpose

- What is the purpose of this evaluation?
- How will findings from the evaluation be used?

Thinking Through a Logic Model

Resources/Inputs
- What resources are available to support the program being evaluated (e.g., staff, money, space, time, partnerships, technology, etc.)?

Activities
- What specific activities are undertaken (or planned) to achieve the outcomes?

Outputs
- What products (e.g., materials, units of services delivered) are produced by your staff as a result of the activities performed?

Outcomes
- What are the program's intended outcomes (intended outcomes are short-term, intermediate, or long-term)?
- What do you ultimately want to change as a result of your activities (long-term outcomes)?
- What occurs between your activities and the point at which you see these ultimate outcomes (short-term and intermediate outcomes)?

Proposed Timeline

- In what timeframe will the evaluation occur?
- When will significant events, such as formal data collection, data analysis, information dissemination, take place?
- Are there any foreseeable bottlenecks or sequencing issues?

Potential Evaluation Budget

- What is the estimated cost for this evaluation?
- Where will the monetary and other resources originate to support the evaluation?

EVALUATION DESIGN

This section provides information on how you will design your evaluation. Provide information on evaluation questions, stakeholder information needs emerging from the evaluation, and the evaluation design.

Evaluation Design
- Which approach do you intend to use to design the program evaluation? (Program-Oriented, Decision-Making, or other? You may research and select another design.)
- Why did you select this design?
- How does the logic model you developed support the selected approach?

Overall Evaluation Goals
- What specific questions do you intend to answer through this evaluation? (State 1-3 questions.)
- Use the SMART goal procedure to formulate 1-3 measurable goals or outcomes for the evaluation aligned to the questions you intend to answer.

DATA COLLECTION

This section provides information on how you will collect/compile data for the proposed evaluation. Provide information on methods by which you will collect/compile data, and how those methods are related to the evaluation questions you identified.

Data Collection
- What data will be collected/compiled to answer the evaluation questions?
- What methods will be used to collect or acquire the data? (e.g., interviews, surveys, questionnaires, existing/secondary data, etc.)
- How will self-evaluation be incorporated into data collection activities?
- From whom or from what will data be collected (source of data)?
- How will the data be protected?

Reliability, Validity, and Ethics
- When selecting your evaluation methodology, how will you address reliability, validity, and ethical considerations?

DATA ANALYSIS & INTERPRETATION

In this section, provide information on indicators and standards you will use to judge success, how you will analyze your evaluation findings, and how you will interpret and justify your conclusions.

Indicators and Standards
- What are some measurable or observable elements that can tell you about the performance of the program being evaluated?
- What constitutes "success"? (i.e., by what standards will you compare your evaluation findings?)

Analysis
- What method will you use to analyze your data?
- Who will you involve in drawing, interpreting, and justifying conclusions?
- What are your plans to involve them in this process?

USE, COMMUNICATION, & EVALUATION

This section provides information about how information from the evaluation plan process and results will be used and shared and how the evaluation itself will be evaluated.

Use
- What actions will be taken to promote evaluation use?

- How will evaluation findings be used?
- Who is responsible for implementing evaluation recommendations?

Communication
- Which evaluation stakeholders will you communicate with and why (e.g., update on status of evaluation, invite to meetings, share interim or final findings)?
- What methods (e.g., in-person meetings, emails, written reports, presentations) will you use to communicate with evaluation stakeholders?
- Why are these methods appropriate for the specific evaluation stakeholder audience of interest?

Evaluating the Evaluation
- How will you evaluate the evaluation? (Instruments? Stakeholder input? Data analysis?)

References
In this section, develop a References page in APA 6th edition format.
Author, A., & Author, B. (date). Title of document. *Journal Title, Volume*(Issue) page-page. doi:######
Author, B., Author, C., & Author, D. D. (n.d.). *Title of document* [Format description]. Retrieved from http://URL

About the Author

Dr. Lisa Marie Portugal holds a PhD in Leadership for Higher Education, an EdD in Public Health Education, a Master of Education in Educational Business Administration – Human Resources, a Master of Education in Health and Wellness, a Master of Arts in Education, and a Bachelor of Fine Arts. She completed 42 credits in a Doctor of Management (DM) in Executive Leadership program. She is a personal and professional life coach, author, university professor, PhD chair, committee member, and a faculty supervisor / mentor to teacher candidates. She currently instructs coursework at the undergraduate, graduate, EdD, and PhD levels for various universities and abroad. She is a researcher, peer-reviewed scholar, and educator. Dr. Portugal is on the review board for various academic journals. Her expertise and research interests include: Virtuous Leadership, Cultural Magnanimity, health and wellness, student engagement and success, student retention, adult learning theory, adult, nontraditional, and at-risk learners, faculty retention, hiring practices, faculty burn-out, best practices in online learning, emerging technology in course design and instruction, online education, learning styles, diversity leadership, and the Community of Inquiry Framework. She integrates theory into practice through conducting research in these areas.

Throughout her career as an educator and mentor, she has taught at 15 universities and abroad. Dr. Portugal has written many books and many peer-reviewed articles in academic and medical journals. She continues to mentor others on how to reach their personal and professional goals, teach online coursework worldwide, research, write, and publish. Dr. Portugal was nominated for the 2020 Celebrity Award Program in the categories of: (1) Fostering an Environment of Diversity and Inclusion; (2) Classroom Performance; (3) Teamwork; (3) Stewardship; (4) Innovation / Creativity; and (5) Professional Contributions. She was nominated for the 2017 Instructional Excellence Award in the Instruction Category.

Dr. Portugal has published research papers in journals such as: Global Journals Incorporated (GJMBR), World Journal of Educational Research, Online Journal of Neurology and Brain Disorders, CPQ Medicine. Cient Periodique, Journal of Natural & Ayurvedic Medicine (JONAM), Archives of General Internal Medicine, Biomedical: Journal of Scientific & Technical Research, Examines in Physical Medicine & Rehabilitation, Diabetes Management, Journal of Instructional Research (JIR), International Journal of Online Pedagogy and Course Design (IJOPCD), Online Journal of Distance Learning Administration (OJDLA), International Journal of Instructional Technology and Distance Learning (ITDL), Academic Leadership the Online Journal, Advancing Women in Leadership Online Journal, Academic Leadership the Online Journal, Online Journal of Distance Learning Administration (OJDLA), and Perspectives on Issues in Higher Education.

Contact

Email:
lisamarieportugal@msn.com

The Leadership Architect
https://drlisamarieportugal.wixsite.com/leadershiparchitect

Website:
http://drlisamarieportugal.weebly.com

Manifest Leadership Academy
https://www.manifestleadershipacademy.com/

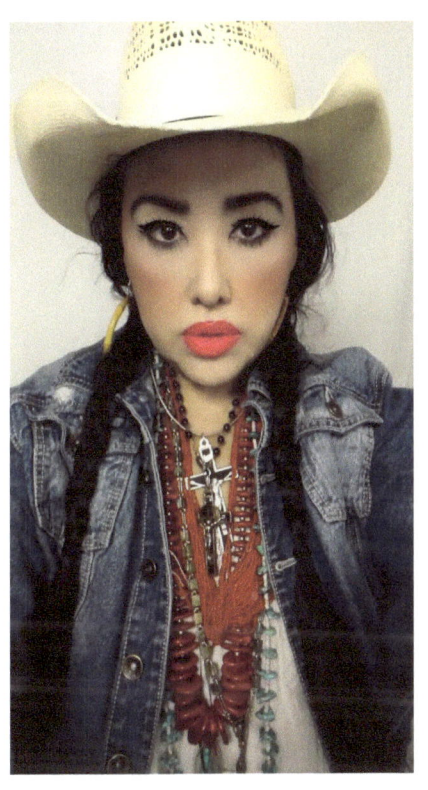

References

American College of Healthcare Executives (ACHE). (2017). About ACHE: ACHE Code of Ethics. Retrieved from http://www.ache.org/ABT_ACHE/code.cfm

Bahous, R., & Nabhani, M. (2011). Assessing education program learning outcomes. Educational Assessment, Evaluation & Accountability, 23(1), 21-39.

Brown, C. A., & McIlroy, K. (2011). Group work in healthcare students' education: What do we think we are doing? Assessment & Evaluation in Higher Education, 36(6), 687-699.

Centers for Disease Control and Prevenation (CDC). (2017, January 19). Division for Heart Disease and Stroke Prevention: Developing and Using a Logic Model. Retrieved from https://www.cdc.gov/dhdsp/programs/spha/evaluation_guides/logic_model.htm

Centers for Disease Control and Prevenation (CDC) (1999, September 17). MMWR: Recommendations and Reports. Retrieved from https://www.cdc.gov/mmwr/preview/mmwrhtml/rr4811a1.htm

Creswell, J.W. (1998). *Qualitative inquiry and research design: Choosing among five traditions.* Thousand Oaks, CA: Sage Publications, Inc.

Decelle, G., & Sherrod, D. (2011). A call to address learner diversity in health professions education. Journal of Best Practices in Health Professions Diversity: Education, Research & Policy, 4(1), 574-584.

Denzin, N. K., & Lincoln, Y. S. (2005). *The Sage handbook of qualitative research.* Thousand Oaks, CA: Sage.

Denzin, N. K., & Lincoln, Y. S., (Eds.). (2012). *Strategies of qualitative research.* Thousand Oaks, CA: Sage.

Dickerson, P. S. (2011). Evaluating an activity: Beyond the 'form.' The Journal of Continuing Education in Nursing, 42(7), 292-293. doi:10.3928/00220124-20110621-02

Dobbin, S. A., & Gatowski, S. I., (1999, March). A Judge's Deskbook on the Basic Philosophies and Methods of Science: Model curriculum [Electronic version]. Retrieved from http://www.unr.edu/bench/chap04.htm

Esposito, E. (2015, November 11). The essential guide to writing S.M.A.R.T. goals. Retrieved from https://www.smartsheet.com/blog/essential-guide-writing-smart-goals

EWTN.news (n.d.). How To Pray the Rosary. Retrieved from https://www.ewtn.com/Devotionals/prayers/rosary/how_to.htm

Fitzpatrick, J. L., Sanders, J. R., & Worthen, B. R. (2004). *Program evaluation: Alternative approaches and practical guidelines* (3rd ed.). Boston: Pearson Education, Inc.

Gall, M. D., Gall, J. P., & Borg, W. R. (2003). *Educational research: An introduction (7th ed.).* Boston, MA: Pearson Education.

Golafshani, N. (2003). Understanding reliability and validity in qualitative research. *The Qualitative Report, 8*(4), 597-607.

Hammersley, M. (1990) *Reading ethnographic research: A critical guide.* London, UK: Longman.

Hays, R. (2009). Assessing learning in primary care. *Education for Primary Care, 20*(1), 4-7.

Hiller, H., & DiLuzio, L. (2004). The interviewee and research interview: Analysing a neglected dimension in research. *Canadian Review of Sociology and Anthropology, 41*(1), 1-26.

Hoepfl, M. C. (1997, Fall). Choosing qualitative research: A primer for technology education researchers. *Journal of Technology Education, 9*(1). Retrieved from http://scholar.lib.vt.edu/ejournals/JTE/v9n1/hoepfl.html

Johnson, B., & Christensen, L. (2008). *Educational research: Quantitative, qualitative, and mixed approaches.* Thousand Oaks, CA: Sage.

Marshall, C., & Rossman, G. (1999) *Designing qualitative research* (3rd ed.). Thousand Oaks, CA: Sage.

McNamara, C. (2007). Basic Guide to Program Evaluation. Retrieved on from http://www.managementhelp.org/evaluatn/fnl_eval.htm

Morell, J. A. (2010, November). Logic Models: Uses, Limitations, Links to Methodology and Data. American Evaluation Association Annual Meeting – San Antonio, TX November 10-13 2010. Retrieved from http://jamorell.com/documents/LM_Workshop_AEA_2010_11_06_2010.pdf

Moustakas, C. (1994). *Phenomenological research methods*. Thousand Oaks, CA: Sage.

Neuman, W. (2003). *Social research methods qualitative and quantitative approaches* (5th ed.). Boston, MA: Allyn and Bacon.

Onwuegbuzie, A. J. & Leech, N. L. (2007, June). Sampling designs in qualitative research: Making the sampling process more public [Electronic version]. *The Qualitative Report, 12*(2), 238-254. Retrieved from http://www.nova.edu/ssss/QR/QR12-2/onwuegbuzie1.pdf

Pincus, H, A., Spaeth-Rublee, B., & Watkins, K. E. (2011, April). The case for measuring quality in mental health and substance abuse care. *Health Affairs, 30*(4). 730-736. doi: 10.1377/hlthaff.2011.0268 Retrieved from http://content.healthaffairs.org/content/30/4/730.full

Portugal, L. M. (2017, July). Educating type 2 diabetes adults about naturopathy, alternative medicine benefits. *Diabetes Management, 7*(3). Retrieved from http://www.openaccessjournals.com/articles/educating-type-2-diabetes-adults-about-naturopathy-alternative-medicine-benefits-12094.html

Portugal, L. M. (2015). *Successful online faculty principles and best practices: Identifiable criteria for employment practices, hiring standards, training, and leadership decisions.* Scholars' Press is a trademark of OmniScriptum GmbH & Co. KG. Saarbrücken, Germany.

Powell, R. R. (2006, Summer). Evaluation research: An overview [Electronic version]. *Library Trends, 55*(1), 102-120.

Rao, V. & Woolcock, M. (2003). Integrating qualitative and quantitative approaches in program evaluation. In F. Bourguignon & F. A. Pereira da Silva (Ed.), *The impact of economic policies on poverty and income distribution: Evaluation techniques and tools* (pp. 165-190). New York, NY: Oxford University Press US.

Roberts, P., & Priest, H. (2006). Reliability and validity in research. *Nursing Standard, 20*, 41-45.

Sanders, J. R. (1994). *The program evaluation standards (2nd ed.)*. Thousand Oaks, CA: Sage Publications, Inc.

Substance Abuse and Mental Health Services Administration (SAMHSA). (2015, June 17). Applying the Strategic Prevention Framework (SPF). Retrieved from https://www.samhsa.gov/capt/applying-strategic-prevention-framework

Substance Abuse and Mental Health Services Administration (SAMHSA). (2016, September 8). Understanding Logic Models. Retrieved from https://www.samhsa.gov/capt/applying-strategic-prevention-framework/step3-plan/understanding-logic-models

Survedi, M. & Morford, S. (2003). Conducting program and project evaluations: A primer for natural resource program managers in British Columbia. *FORREX—Forest Research Extension Partnership, Kamloops, B.C. FORREX Series 6.*

The Electoral Knowledge Network: ACE. (2017). Civic and Voter Education. Retrieved from https://aceproject.org/ace-en/topics/ve/veh/veh03/veh03e

University of Virginia: Employee Development. (n.d.). Writing S.M.A.R.T. goals. Retrieved from http://www.hr.virginia.edu/uploads/documents/media/Writing_SMART_Goals.pdf

Walker, W. (2007). Ethical considerations in phenomenological research. *Nurse Researcher, 14*(3), 36-45.

Wilde, J. & Sockey, S. (1995, December). Evaluation handbook [Electronic version]. *EAC West, New Mexico Highlands University*. Retrieved from http://www.ncela.gwu.edu/pubs/eacwest/evalhbk.htm

Young, C. (2007). Blending qualitative and quantitative methods for program evaluation: The application and insights of the exit interview [Electronic version]. Retrieved from http://74.125.45.132/search?q=cache:RxBseUaBojMJ:www.apsanet.org/tlc2007/TLC07Young.pdf+Qualitative+Approaches+to+Program+Evaluation&hl=en&ct=clnk&cd=17&gl=us

Young, R. A., Roberts, R. G., & Holden, R. J. (2017). The challenges of measuring, improving, and reporting quality in primary care. *Annals of Family Medicine, 15*(2), 175-182. doi:10.1370/afm.2014

Disclaimer: The content of this book is based on research conducted by Dr. Lisa Marie Portugal, unless otherwise noted. The information is presented for educational purposes only and is not intended to diagnose or prescribe for any condition, nor to prevent, treat, mitigate or cure such conditions. The information contained herein is not intended to replace a one–on–one relationship with a qualified professional. Therefore, this information is not intended as advice, but rather a sharing of knowledge and information based on research and experience. This book and Dr. Lisa Marie Portugal encourages you to make your own decisions based on your judgment and research. The information in this book is not intended to diagnose, treat, cure, or prevent any problem. I am not diagnosing, prescribing, advising, or practicing. I am merely presenting information for you to review, research, and consider. In addition, I receive no money or endorse any products or services listed in this book. Seek professional advice and service from your sources. You and only you are responsible if you choose to do anything based on what you read.

www.ingramcontent.com/pod-product-compliance
Lightning Source LLC
Chambersburg PA
CBHW040217220526
45473CB00001B/15